Vagus Nerve Unlocked

Guide to Unleashing Your Self-healing Ability and Achieving Freedom from Anxiety, Depression, PTSD, Trauma, Inflammation, and Autoimmunity

Table of contents

Vagus Nerve Unlocked

INTRODUCTION

Researchers will know that feeling, the small euphoria of that "eureka" moment when a person finds that everything he has studied so far fits together like some splendid jigsaw puzzle. That was what I felt when I first discovered the existence of the vagus nerve.

Let me back track a bit. I had always had some interest in the study of diseases, and how they form. I know that the human body is a massive interconnected network of organs and feedback systems, even as it is also connected to the outside world. I was thinking, "what if it is possible to boil down the causes of a lot of diseases into a smaller set of factors?" Sure, we already have things like diet, lifestyle, genetics, and the like. What if it could be further narrowed down? I was going for something like an amateur's version of the Grand Unified Field Theory, only this time related to the formation of diseases.

So I read, researched, even took a few courses to understand what I was reading. In the course of my study, I found a word that has been mentioned in passing in various literature:

"Vagus nerve"

Here it mentions that the disease affects the vagus nerve. There it mentions that the effects can be seen in the vagus nerve. Another research paper claims that managing the vagus nerve could help calm the symptoms of the disease I was looking up at the time.

Now, I wouldn't have paid much attention, had it not been for the fact that I saw the word in absolutely different types of research papers. I saw it pretty prominently in research on epilepsy, then in passing on a paper about the good effects of lactobacilli in the gut. I saw it again on a study on cardiovascular illnesses, and then once more in pulmonary injuries. I was intrigued. It was like seeing an Easter egg appear here and there, a vaguely familiar factor that keeps persisting. So I did what any sane man would do: I Googled.

And that's when the floodgates opened.

Somehow, everything I studied in the past came together in the image of a bundle of nerve fibers.

A New Focal Point

Science, like the media, likes to have its darlings. In the field of technology and gadgets, for example, engineers are struggling to fit more and more computing power in as small a space as possible. In the field of rocket science, physicists are perpetually trying to break records of payload and fuel efficiency.

In the field of medicine... well, the darlings can be quite numerous. That's partly because the discipline is broken down into a huge number of smaller ones, each one trying to pursue a different thread that when woven together hopefully brings us better health.

But there are times when these disciplines bump into each other in discovery, as they find common ground. These are the focal points of health, and they are of great interest when they appear because they represent a single factor that has the ability to influence a massive host of other factors. The DNA was such a focal point when it was discovered and eventually mapped. Before the DNA, the discovery of the cell was a huge focal point.

Now, as I found, the discovery of the vagus nerve and its various implications appear to be the next big focal point in the field of health.

What is it to you?

You're probably wondering now why you should spend your time going over this "vagus nerve". I'll answer this one up front — this might be the biggest health-related idea you have come across with in forever, and you would want to know just how the proper stimulation of this nerve could improve your daily life. I won't be exaggerating when I say that this could change your future, with regards to your health. With this knowledge, you can avoid a landmine of possible health issues, and even turn back the hands of time to resolve illnesses that have already taken hold. I won't even be exaggerating when I say that knowledge of the vagus nerve can *literally* affect the welfare of the future generation! You'll see that in shocking detail at the last part of this book.

These pages are the culmination of my lengthy study on the concept of the vagus nerve, and the various health factors that it influences. I tried my best to make complicated medical information as accessible as possible, even as I explore various theories. I also did my best to make the book as practical as possible, so that you can have takeaways that you can also share to others. Within these pages, you will find not just theories and results of various studies, but also a generous helping of self-care tips you can then use at *any* moment. I know you're investing precious time reading this book, so I strived to make the knowledge presented as easy to apply as possible, while not compromising on the impact it could bring to your life.

So strap in, and prepare for a wealth of cutting-edge knowledge about your health and how you can improve it! Believe me when I say that all it takes is a few deep breaths and soothing touches — but what you will learn before you get to that conclusion will blow your mind!

PART 1:

The Basics

CHAPTER 1: The Vagus Nerve: A Tale of Many Cities

"New roads; new ruts." -- Gilbert K. Chesterton

The human body may be one of the most precious things Nature has ever created. It is a complex array of organs and cells, each one with specialization, and yet each one dependent on each other to survive. While some might argue the case of animals and other creatures with much more complex structures, the human body is unique simply because it is the only one endowed with as much brain power.

And, while it's still debatable, this brain power stands at the very core of what humanity is all about. Our ability to grow and evolve, to learn and to plan, to invent and to theorize, to do high-order cognitive tasks, all reside in our brains. Our brains allowed us to progress from caves and trees to the creation of virtual realities.

But while the brain is amazing, it would be completely useless without its supporting cast. Every organ, every system, has at least some role that relates to the protection of the brain. The rest of the nervous system, for example, consists of pathways for signals to travel from the brain to other parts of the body.

And this is where it gets interesting. The brain would be an isolated city of ultimate complexity if it were not connected by the "roads" that are the neural network. Can you imagine a world where each city, prosperous as they are, would be isolated from each other because of the lack of connections? That wouldn't be much of a world. In history, the creation of roads and other transport routes have been one of the greatest catalysts of progress. The human body, too, has many great cities -- but what truly defines them is how they are connected to each other.

In the body, there are set "roads" that travel to other "cities" in the body, sending instructions on how they can make the body better as a whole. But two sets of roads stand out from all others.

One of them is the spinal cord, essentially an extension of the brain, a superhighway through which the brain sends signals to other parts of the body. Break this superhighway, and the brain ceases to have control over motion and other voluntary functions. The function of the spinal cord is very well-known, and has been subjected to much study.

But there is another superhighway in the body that isn't as popular, but could be just as important. This one does not lead to the voluntary muscles that power the body's movement. Rather, this one is connected to some extremely important and sensitive organs -- the heart, the lungs, and the stomach to name a few.

This nerve actually connects the core of life. Take out one of these organs, and the whole body dies. In contrast, some people have been known to live through spinal cord damage (albeit with debilitating effects). Indeed, it would be possible to lose function in some parts of the spinal cord and still live, while significant loss of function in this other superhighway of nerves would mean an agonizing death. The implications of this nerve's connections has pretty recently seized the attention of researchers as a possible answer to many health issues. Many have considered this to be the holy grail of modern medicine — a panacea that could end a host of modern diseases with minimal effort.

Enter the Vagus Nerve

What if I tell you that there is a single bundle of nerves in your body that controls your whole well-being? You would probably be laughing now, but it actually exists.

onsider this. A single, overpowered nerve bundle has the power to control such diverse aspects of your personality as:

- Heart rate
- Memory

- Breathing

- Healing

- Relaxation

- Hunger and satiation

- Emotion

This may be a very short list, but what a diverse list it is! You can immediately see how this nerve, called the vagus nerve, can have an incredible impact on your life.

The Hard Science

The vagus nerve goes by many names. In the olden days, it was called the "pneumogastric nerve" due to the way it connects the brain and the lungs, and the stomach. Another designation is "CN X", or Cranial Nerve X. Despite being a paired bundle, it is commonly described as a singular nerve. As such, it is the longest nerve of our autonomic nervous system. This is that part of the nervous system that controls the "autonomic" processes of the smooth muscles and the various glands, thus having a vital role in our body's function and development.

The name "vagus" came about when physicians realized that the nerve takes a "wandering" course throughout the body. It is literally a wandering nerve, coming from the skull and making its way down towards the abdominal cavity. The word "vagus" is also the root of the word "vagabond".

In the past, the vagus nerve was simply thought of as that nerve that connects various important parts of the body, helping them function. Today, however, more of its unique and fascinating functions have been uncovered.

Vagus Nerve Structure

The vagus nerve is what is called a "mixed nerve", a nerve that is composed of both "efferent" (signal-sending) and "afferent" (signal-receiving or sensory) fibers. The vagus is about 20% efferent and 80% afferent, which is important because this combination allows it to effectively communicate with a huge group of organs. Most of the other nerves in the autonomic nervous system is efferent, since they are mostly used to control other parts of the body. But the afferent qualities of the vagus nerve allows not just for control but also for a feedback mechanism. This way, the brain (on the other end of the nerve) doesn't just tell the body to start or stop a certain process. The body can also tell the brain more about the status of the process, whether it has been started or completed, and what potential issues may have arose from the performance of the process.

The vagus nerve stems from the base of the brain (the brainstem), going down through the neck, the chest, and down to the abdominal section. As the nerve traverses this line, it also has several branches that touch various organs such as the pharynx, larynx, lungs, heart, and the gastrointestinal tract. In the brain, the ends of the nerve are connected to other important regions including the amygdala, hypothalamus, and thalamus.

Stimulating the Vagus Nerve

Because it is so expansive, the vagus nerve can be accessed ("stimulated") in a wide variety of ways. Its first recorded roots (at least, if we go by medical records) reaches back to the 1880s, when it was found that manually massaging and compressing the carotid artery in the neck's cervical region could help suppress seizures. This was the first time medical professionals attributed the stimulation (albeit a crude one) of the vagus nerve to the suppression of seizures. In the 1930s and the 1940s, the electrical stimulation of the vagus nerve was experimented on, to understand the influence of this segment of the autonomic nervous system and in the electrical activity of the brain. Animal experimentation determined that the nerve had a role to play in other types of brain activity. Later, it was confirmed that the vagus nerve plays an important role in the treatment of convulsion (though the relationship was first reached when experimenting with dogs, and not with human samples).

After this, the connection of the vagus nerve to the diaphragm was established. This was when deep breathing and paced breathing were both considered effective means to influence the mind through the vagus nerve. The nerve's connection to both the heart and lungs had been postulated to be among the reasons why there is a positive cognitive and emotional stimulation when we do cardio-respiratory exercises. In fact, ancient exercise like yoga and breathing techniques had been thought to be effective partly because of this same connection.

A time passed, dedicated experiments had been approved by the US FDA in order to determine other possible benefits of vagal stimulation. The first implanted device meant to stimulate the nerve was put into service in 1997. This was meant to treat refractory epilepsy. This device was itself later FDA approved, ushering in the era of further research on the benefits of vagus nerve stimulation. It is interesting to know, though, that the device didn't get the FDA certification as an epilepsy cure -- it was meant to help treat chronic treatment-resistant depression! This was also around the time doctors started understanding more about the role of the vagus nerve in the nurturing of mental well-being.

From depression, research quickly moved to other psychological conditions such as bipolar disorder and anxiety disorders. Other brain-related issues, from chronic headaches to Alzheimer's, also got the vagus nerve stimulation treatment. From there, researchers have started moving into lifestyle issues, such as obesity. While the body of literature on these subjects show some promise, none of them are as of yet definitive and hence none are yet FDA-approved. But just looking at this history shows that this bundle of nerve fibers shows much potential for improving not just a specific group of conditions, but also our entire wellbeing.

Measuring Vagus Health: Heart Rate Variability

Science lives on measurement, and something does not exist unless it can be concretely measured. Throughout this book, you will encounter nearly-unbelievable accounts of how much the vagus nerve can affect several areas of your life -- literally, the wellbeing of your mind, body, and spirit rests in this long bundle of nerves. But before that, we need to know just how you can measure whether your vagus nerve is doing well or not.

As we are talking about something that is deeply embedded in the body, the surest way to measure vagus nerve health is by sticking instruments into your neck and back and measuring the minuscule impulses that travel through your vagus nerve as your body responds to different stimuli. But that's like saying you can only measure your heart rate by getting a monitor to observe the beating of your heart. For a body part this vital and well-connected, there must be an easier way.

Since the vagus nerve's health cannot be measured in size and mass like muscles, or in visible functioning like organs, scientists have created a benchmark to measure how well the vagus nerve performs. This wellbeing is termed "vagal tone", and the benchmark is called "heart rate variability".

Heart Rate Variability (HRV) is, simply put, the time difference between heartbeats. It is the interval between one beat and another, and can be read on the electrocardiogram as the RR variability, which refers to the R waves that correspond to the depolarization of the ventricles. These measures have been found to correlate to the healthy balance between the sympathetic and parasympathetic nervous systems, and has been confirmed in empirical studies.

Further research has found that HRV has been correlated to the mortality rate of different diseases. For example, studies as early as 50 years ago have revealed that HRV marked the possible onset of fetal distress even before there had been actual, measurable changes in the heart rate. Today, HRV has been found to be a good indicator for various syndrome and diseases.

How does this relate to the vagus nerve? Since the vagus nerve is attached to the heart, and therefore plays a role in its contractions, it has been found that a weakening in the vagus nerve can actually be the root cause in the heightening of disease mortality rates. These correlations become even more manifest when a medical procedure has been done which may have touched or damaged the vagus nerve's heart connection, such as cardiac surgery. HRV can also be a determinative factor in predicting the severity of conditions such as rheumatoid arthritis, some autoimmune diseases, and even bowel diseases.

These findings also come in contrast to the previous idea that it was these diseases that cause a decrease in the vagus nerve activity. For some time it was taught that diseases caused a concomitant neural damage, weakening the vagus. It has since then been found to be the other way around. This is especially pronounced in diseases that cause inflammation. Since the vagus nerve is also an important part of the anti-inflammatory circuit of the nervous system, what would have been normal inflammatory responses become aggravated because of the weakened vagus nerve.

Further studies have established the vagus nerve as the "grand central station" of nerve pathways where the most important functions of the body meet. Without specialized (and highly intrusive) equipment, it would be impossible to tell just how well the vagus nerve is functioning. Our best, and scientifically proven bet is Heart Rate Variability, which is the most readily available indicator to measure how well one of the most important bundle of nerves in the body is doing its job.

Takeaways:

- The vagus nerve is responsible for a huge array of bodily processes.

- The vagus nerve's health is important, and it can be measured through heart rate variability.

CHAPTER 2: Fighting the Undefined: The Secret Powers of the Vagus Nerve

*"**Now comes the mystery.**"* -- Henry Ward Beecher

Hopefuls in the scientific and medical community have long been looking for that silver bullet of health that can destroy the many health issues that have plagued man. It's not a new endeavor, either -- the alchemists of old have spent their lives (and massive resources) looking for the Elixir of Life. In the modern day, science keeps on discovering new and interesting ideas that inch us closer to that panacea. Among these is the vagus nerve.

There are many reasons why the vagus nerve has become a fairly hot topic recently. Recent research has proven that the vagus nerve not only touches several organs in the body, but also several aspects of life that we thought are simply too abstract or too difficult to be directly addressed.

Think, for example, the concepts of rampant weight gain (or difficulty of weight loss), depression, and inflammation. The common denominator among these is the fact that all of them are multifaceted issues that are usually addressed by medication and therapy. But these medication and therapy approaches usually attempt to cure only the overt symptoms of the issue, while only rarely being able to go down deep enough to cure their roots.

Yes, these issues can be caused by a very wide variety of factors. Weight gain, for example, can be as much a lifestyle issue as it can be a problem of genetics or a physiological illness. Depression can be caused by a chemical imbalance, and it can also be a direct product of a toxic and repressive environment. Inflammation can be due to any damage, ranging from an injury to an infection. And yet, all of these issues have something to do with the way the brain interfaces with the body, where the brain causes reactions in the body sent through -- you guessed it -- the vagus nerve and similar nerve systems.

Recent research has found out that these three issues, otherwise undefined (or very roughly so) can be eased by activating the vagus nerve. This is among the many secret powers of the vagus nerve that most people are yet to discover.

Let's take a look at how the vagus nerve specifically relates to these issues.

Vagus Nerve and Weight Problems

Obesity is something that is almost a given in today's world. It is a rampant concern, made worse by today's sedentary, tech-oriented lifestyle and fast-food-first diet. We already know that obesity is a major factor in several lifestyle diseases, such as hypertension and diabetes. An obese person is also much more likely to die from stroke or heart attack.

Despite the many factors that surround obesity, science has found it undeniable that the whole idea of weight gain and weight loss is mediated in great part by the activity of the vagus nerve. The idea of using this connection to treat weight loss was first floated when a study found that depressed people who used vagus nerve stimulation devices also reported weight loss, completely independent from the improvement (or lack thereof) of their depressive states. These improvements prove that the vagus nerve acts a mediator of weight gain or loss independent of its effects on the psyche.

The vagus nerve is the one that mediates the signals of hunger and satiety. When you eat, the expansion in your stomach triggers the sending of signals to your brain saying you are already full. When your gut changes that there has been a change in the nourishment of your body, it can also start sending either hunger or satiety signals to the brain.

While the causes of obesity are different, researchers have found that most people who are obese also suffer from a lower sensitivity of the vagus nerve. This means that it cannot immediately relay the satiety signals from the stomach to the brain. When this happens, the person continues eating as if he was still hungry, stopping only when the signals are finally sent to the brain.

This insensitivity isn't caused by obesity per se. In fact, the food we eat is more likely to blame. A 2016 study has found that many food items that induce obesity are also responsible for reducing vagus nerve sensitivity at the same time. The same study has also found that the vagus nerve can be used as a treatment target for obesity. Current techniques used have resulted in a mixed bag of results for human studies, but research is still ongoing.

Aside from mediating the feeling of satiation, it has also been proven that a healthy vagus nerve can help reduce cravings. Vagus nerve stimulation is also more sustainable as a means of treatment, since the results have found that the loss of weight is proportional to the excess weight.

Later in this book, we will be looking at the different ways on how vagus nerve stimulation can be done, but right now, there are two opposing approaches to using the vagus nerve as a treatment staging point for obesity. First, there is the natural method of just stimulating the vagus nerve, in an attempt to make it more sensitive in transmitting the signals from your stomach to your brain. Then, there is also the method of blocking (or regulating) the activity of the vagus nerve, by bypassing the natural signal sending of the stomach and instead sending artificial signals to the brain.

The latter technique is done through an implanted device that interfaces with the vagus nerve. We will read more about these implants in a later chapter on electronic stimulation, but for now suffice it to say that such an implant (FDA-approved) can be placed through a minimally-invasive procedure. The device senses the stomach's activity, and sense satiety signals through the vagus nerve as soon as it detects that the stomach has received food. In effect, it dupes the brain into thinking that you are already full after just a few bites.

This is currently being looked at as an alternative to the more common obesity treatment that is gastric bypass, which aims to force the stomach into reducing its capacity, therefore sending satiety signals early. The advantage of the vagus nerve stimulator is that it is reversible, and therefore there is no danger of causing malnutrition or runaway weight loss.

Vagus Nerve and Depression

It has been predicted that by 2030, depression would be the second most dangerous disease humanity will face, only right after HIV. Unless science finds out exactly how depression develops so it could create a cure, the current social conditions seem to still point to this bleak future.

The vagus nerve has also been studied as the ideal treatment location for depression, specifically treatment-resistant depression. This is the type of depression that can no longer be treated by medication and therapy. This is actually a significant number, as it is noted that two out of three patients who suffer from major depressive problems do not benefit from the first prescriptions given by doctors. One third of all patients, on the other hand, do not respond to any prescription at all. In response, the FDA has approved vagus nerve stimulation devices for the treatment of depression back in 2005.

Depression treatment via the vagus nerve takes the form of "hacking" the brain -- this means attaching a device for electronic vagus stimulation, which delivers impulses directly affecting the part of the brain that affects the mood. Some experts also hypothesize that stimulating the vagus nerve in this way helps increase one's sense of focus, which is markedly one of the things lost during depressive episodes. After the surgery to implant the device, a person can feel alert and relaxed enough to resume normal physical, social, and emotional functioning. This may sound like pretty invasive procedure, but it is actually pretty safe and trials have produced a mainly positive result, especially when combined with traditional methods. Some studies have found that around half of test subjects responded favorably to vagus nerve stimulation, though around 40% of them relapsed soon after when the stimulation was stopped or removed.

Another way in which such devices help the depressed individual is by what is known as the "anti-convulsive effect", where the stimulation acts as an anticonvulsant system (similar to how it prevents the onset of epileptic seizures) to help relieve depressive symptoms. This is analogous to the use of some antidepressant drugs such as lamotrigine and carbamazepine, which are all also anticonvulsive.

Perhaps even more powerfully, the vagus nerve activation can cause changes in the local anatomy of the brain. The nerve has ends that are connected to the part that regulates mood, and some neurologists have hypothesized that stimulation can change how these areas of the brain work over prolonged periods of time.

Another way that the vagus nerve helps to reduce depressive episodes is in its regulation of the neurotransmitters noradrenaline and 5-hydroxytryptamine. These two substances are reduced during cases of depression, and some medications work to ensure that the brain has enough supply of these two neurotransmitters. It is believed that the vagus nerve, when activated, does the same.

One thing to remember, though, is that electronic VNS stimulation for depression treatment is not a quick treatment. In fact, it can take months (up to 9 months has been reported) before the effects can be felt. This is why one needs to practice conventional methods in tandem with electronic stimulation, in order to maintain one's welfare in between the start of treatment and the effect.

The side effects reported for this type of VNS is similar to the usual side effects reported for all types of electronic stimulation. This will be explored in detail later. The biggest issue with this type of treatment is the continuous operation of the pulse-emitting device. The battery will have to be replaced every now and then, and the operation needed for this would expose the patient to risk of infection. Still, this is an acceptable trade-off as the device can greatly enhance one's wellbeing.

Vagus Nerve and Anxiety

As alluded to in the previous section, one can gain reprieve from (often random) bouts of anxiety thanks to vagus nerve stimulation. Among the many signals carried by this superhighway of nerves are signals that relate to calm and nervousness, anger, and relaxation. This is tied to the vagus nerve's connection to the heart and lungs -- two organs that get really overworked when exposed to increased levels of anxiety.

An insensitive vagus nerve could fail to quickly perform its task of stopping the sympathetic nervous system from continuously sending signals. A person who is anxious engages this part of the nervous system, stimulating a fight-or-flight response. The vagus nerve, along with the rest of the parasympathetic nervous system, is charged with ceasing this response when the danger has passed (or, as the case may be, when there really is no dangers at all). When this happens, the sympathetic nervous system takes over the body, being able to send stress signals at will even when not necessary. This imbalance is at the root of most panic attacks. It also creates a vicious circle -- when the body is stressed, it creates more glutamate, which is a chemical that can provoke even more anxiety. This results in a host of physical issues, ranging from irritability and irrationality when making decisions to migraine, insomnia, and other health issues. It also hampers the formation of new memories, thanks to a reduced volume in the hippocampus (the part of the brain that facilitates the formation of memories).

Because the vagus is insensitive, anxiety has also been widely known to trigger discomfort in many of the organs facilitated by the nerve. This includes issues with the gastrointestinal tract (anywhere from hyperacidity to contractions) as well as difficulty in breathing and irregular heartbeats.

The good news is that you don't need an implant in order to control vagus nerve issues arising from (and causing more) anxiety. The usual natural methods, from deep breathing to the practice of enjoyable physical activities, can greatly help remedy the issue. This vagus nerve connection is the primary reason why such relaxation techniques, from deep breathing to the more advanced forms, have become so successful even since the olden times of yoga and such.

Perhaps even more interestingly, the vagus nerve has also been pointed to as essential in the enhancement of what psychologists call "extinction learning". Extinction learning is the term used when a person is exposed to a fear or anxiety-generating stimuli over and over again, until such time that he (and his mind) realizes that the stimuli does not carry any inherent danger. This effectively makes the fear extinct. Vagus nerve stimulation applied at the same time has been said to greatly increase the extinction process. Research done on this avenue has also tangentially produced results that point to the role of the vagus nerve in the formation of memory, and scientists are also exploring the fact that the vagus nerve may also be hacked to help a person remember things more easily! Such undefined factors as anxiety, fear, and memory are all vastly affected by the vagus nerve.

Vagus Nerve and Trauma

Trauma is often a touchy topic, arguably as much as (if not even more so than) depression. Deep psychological trauma such as that caused by extreme periods of stress or emotional states can greatly contribute to the downward spiral of a person. This is not the type of mental issue that can be treated just so by medications -- it needs a more personal, therapeutic approach. Aside from counseling, those who have undergone extreme bouts of trauma have been taught to practice meditation and other mindfulness techniques (incidentally, all practices that help stimulate the vagus nerve). But even then, these may not be enough.

Stimulating the vagus nerve, though, through concrete methods (short of electronic stimulation) can help improve one's trauma management and is essential in reinforcing the results of various therapeutic techniques. As we will see later, stimulating the vagus nerve is essential in increasing its connectivity, therefore improving the body's rest-and-digest system in order to let it recuperate. A good vagus nerve connection helps improve the natural stress management system of the body, and also helps reduce the brain's overreaction to stimuli.

A group of Swiss scientists have found out that the afferent bundle of the vagus nerve is directly related to how the body handles response to fear and anxiety. The Swiss research found that a healthy vagus nerve (measured through vagal tone) can help overcome one's conditioned fears -- a fact that is of great importance to people whose primary source of trauma is a fearful encounter, such as war veterans and people with PTSD. In the study, it was found that a healthy vagus nerve slows down the fear-related response from the body (specifically, the gut) to the brain, therefore preventing spikes from the sympathetic nervous system. The researchers have also tried blocking these signals altogether, and they found that this induced a longer retention of "learned" fears.

This is especially important for PTSD patients, as a healthy and stimulated vagus nerve can help re-associate stimuli from a person's surroundings. Stimuli that had once been associated with threatening situations can be reinterpreted to mean safer surroundings. The efficacy of direct vagus nerve stimulation to induce this state is still being studied, but current findings are very illuminating. As the researchers put it, it is remarkable how altering a simple signal path from the gut to the brain can result in complex changes in one's behavior.

Vagus Nerve and Epilepsy

One of the first therapeutic applications of vagus nerve stimulation has been done in the field of epileptic seizures. It is also one of the places where vagus nerve stimulation has become highly successful. Today, VNS devices and stimulation techniques have been the answer to epileptic cases that do not respond to medications (drug-resistant epilepsy).

The weird thing is that research has not defined exactly how stimulation stops the onset of epileptic seizures. We do know that epilepsy is caused by runaway electric signals in the brain, "shocking" the body into seizures. Regular, mild pulses sent through the vagus nerve does not really help disrupt these signals, but other mechanisms have been put forward. One is the fact that stimulation helps increase the blood flow to key areas in the brain, making them more resistant or less prone to seizure attacks. The process also raises some levels of neurotransmitters that control seizures, therefore increasing the body's natural ability to prevent these seizures on its own. It is also suggested that the regular pulses which the stimulation device emits helps change the overall EEG patterns during a seizure, preventing these effects.

The latest models of the stimulation devices have harnessed an additional dimension of the vagus nerve's connection to the brain. Research has found that around 80% of all people who experience seizures also experience heightened heart rate before the seizure begins. Newer devices can pick these heart rate changes, allowing the machine to provide an extra burst of pulses to prevent the seizure from even forming.

It is important to understand that vagus nerve stimulation is merely an add-on to existing epilepsy treatment methods, and not a standalone treatment -- unless in the express condition that the epilepsy is not treatable by any other type of medication.

Before being lined up for vagus nerve stimulator implantation, the person is first screened. First, physicians have to make sure that the cause of the seizure is epileptic, and not some other issue. Stimulation will only help if the seizures are caused by runaway electric activity in the brain. Some research have found that generalized epileptic seizures can also be improved by vagus nerve stimulation, but most of the curative results have been focused on focal seizures.

It is also important to test out and exhaust all other avenues for treatment. For example, the lack of effect by medications does not necessarily mean that the epilepsy is drug-resistant -- it can be a lifestyle issues, where the patient has difficulty taking the medications on time and regularly. There may also be other behavior affecting the intensity of the seizures, such as poor nutritional choices. A physician will first make sure that the appropriate medicines (different ones for different seizure types) are taken at the appropriate times and durations.

All these checks are done to ensure that vagus nerve stimulation will work as intended, as it can be dangerous for a person be installed with a stimulation device when the seizure is caused by different reasons. Because of possible side effects, a person undergoing non-epileptic seizures can, for example, have difficulty breathing at the same time, or may have his heart slow down or speed up at the same time. Combined, these factors could be very harmful. Follow ups are also made after the device installation, to adjust the intensity as needed.

The very first vagus nerve stimulation implant done on a human being was performed in 1988. This was way before the FDA approved the use of such devices for cure in cases of epilepsy. Further studies show that the later generations of such implants were so successful that they reduced the seizures by around 50% for the first year. This has increased to more than 64% in later studies.

Vagus Nerve and Brain Growth

It has been thought, long ago, that the brain does not grow new neurons during adulthood. However, new research has shown that there are parts of the brain that continued to grow even during later life, through a process called neurogenesis. This is especially pronounced in certain areas, and it has also been found that vagus nerve stimulation helps greatly in this growth. This knowledge is especially useful when one considers the case of people who have undergone brain operations. Long-term vagus nerve stimulation can cause a continued increase in the number of new brain cells persisting even if the stimulation is discontinued for some time.

This effect is directly brought about by the same mechanism that reduces depression through the vagus nerve. It has been found that increased levels of noradrenalin can increase the production of new cells in the hippocampal region. It has also been found that the stimulation of the production of serotonin helps in the same neurogenetic activity. This is connected to the fact that, in the past, studies have shown that anti-depressant drugs have actually helped trigger neurogenesis even in adults. It all boils down to the increased activity in the sites that produce the relevant neurotransmitters.

Vagus Nerve and Sleep Disorders

Because of the vagus nerve's important role in the rest-and-digest system, it also plays an important role in maintaining one's health during sleep. While it does not actually put the body to sleep, it plays a vital role in maintaining the other bodily functions that allow the body to function well when all conscious control is gone.

When the vagus nerve fails in this function, sleep disorders may occur. One of them is obstructive sleep apnea, which is a breathing disorder that causes the inability to breathe while asleep. As breathing is regulated by the vagus nerve, physicians have found that vagus nerve stimulation is also instrumental in resolving sleep apnea issues. To further highlight just how vital the vagus nerve is, it is also to be noted that sleep apnea is a concern that usually appears along with epilepsy.

Sleep apnea, obviously, causes difficulty sleeping. Even worse, it starts a downward spiral as the vagus nerve (and the whole parasympathetic nervous system it is a part of) can be greatly harmed by lack of sleep. The parasympathetic system is a part of a two-way system, and it activates best when its complement (the sympathetic axis formed by the hypothalamus, pituitary gland, and adrenal glands) is at rest. Sleeplessness causes this part of the nervous system to remain alert for extended periods of time, thus undermining the activity of the vagus nerve. This then contributes to other health problems, such as hypertension and weight gain. You may want to dial back on your caffeine intake to allow your body to rest some more. Sleep issues arising from other conditions, like insomnia, also has to be taken care of separately in order to ensure good vagus nerve health. While there are several possible causes for sleep disorders, from the physical to the psychological, there are corresponding treatments for all of them that you can look into to prevent further damage to your health.

Vagus Nerve, Inflammation, and Pain

In today's world, pain seems to be a constant companion, so much that painkillers and analgesics seem to be a part of everyday life. Technology has coerced us into working for extended hours without moving, a sedentary lifestyle that leads to chronic pain issues. Even those who workout daily and live a healthy lifestyle aren't exempt from the pain -- a single wrong lift, a few wrong movements, and you can bust a part of your body leading again to chronic pain.

The vagus nerve is, again, linked to how the body processes pain and inflammation. In fact, research on this subject has been one of the first clues that scientifically linked the vagus nerve to many of the processes now attributed to its functions. In the late 1990s, a New York-based neurosurgeon discovered that when an anti-inflammatory drug was injected into a rat's brain, the drug had the unusual effect of blocking inflammation elsewhere in the rat's body. This was despite the fact that the dosage injected was far too small to be carried into the bloodstream, to affect the other cells. During further research, he realized that the vagus nerve was responsible for carrying the anti-inflammatory signals from the brain to other parts of the body. This became the basis for future research on how the vagus nerve can help turn off pain and inflammation in other parts of the body. It was also the first actual proof that the brain and the nervous system is inextricably linked to the various organs of our body and their cells, not only regulating their functions but also their wellbeing.

The vagus nerve carries immune signals to the rest of the body. This is why it has also been studied as a treatment point for inflammatory diseases such as arthritis. It has been pointed out earlier that arthritis is also one of the diseases whose worsening can be predicted by HRV or Heart Rate Variability. In more recent studies, it has been found that aside from the brain using the vagus nerve to spread out immune signals, the brain also uses the vagus nerve to detect the overall state of the body's immune system, thus allowing the core of the nervous system to regulate its response. These studies have also begun looking into just which cytokines (proteins that mediate the interactions between the body's cells) produce which effect in the vagus nerve, possibly ushering in a new era of pain treatment and management.

Inflammation is not all about pain, too. In fact, inflammation is an immune response that could take different forms. For example, it can cause an upset stomach, or even histamine-induced itching. This is an important finding, because there are some medications for these same conditions that actually counteract how the vagus nerve naturally works to cure these illnesses. For example, there are certain medications that block the production and use of acetylcholine, which is how the vagus nerve communicates to the rest of the body. When taking medications for issues that can be connected to the vagus nerve, it is best to ask your doctor for more natural (or at least vagus-friendly) alternatives.

The idea that stimulating the vagus nerve (either naturally or through electronic alternatives) is a key element in preventing pain and inflammation has also been a major thrust of the new field called "bioelectronic integrative medicine". This field looks into how issues that used to be treated with medication (such as pain and inflammation, with analgesics) could be better aided by the use of neuromodulation devices. The use of implants and other vagus nerve stimulation techniques have been found to be effective in keeping the symptoms of pain and inflammation at bay, but for now science is still not able to permanently remove these symptoms. Stop the stimulation, and the symptoms resume. In the future, advances in the field could make pain and inflammation a thing of the past.

Vagus Nerve and Hypertension

Even if you are already hypertensive, you might not know that there are actually different types of hypertension depending on where the elevated blood pressure is. A specific type, for example, is Pulmonary Hypertension, where there is increased blood pressure in the pulmonary vasculature. Like other types of hypertension, it can cause a wide variety of accompanying diseases. A subclass of Pulmonary Hypertension, Pulmonary Artery Hypertension, is especially lethal with half of all diagnosed patients dying within seven years from their initial diagnosis.

Pulmonary Hypertension is complex, and it is very difficult to trace the interplay between the various cells and systems of the body leading to the illness and its effects. One thing for certain, however, is that the vagus nerve has a huge role to play in this illness. This knowledge, only recently studied in detail, comes in stark contrast with the way that Pulmonary Hypertension has been usually treated. In the past, it has been alleviated by efforts to inhibit the activity of the sympathetic nervous system, usually through medications. A more potent alternative, instead, is the restoration of balance through the activation of the vagus nerve, and along with it the rest of the parasympathetic nervous system.

In experiments with animal subjects, it has been found that stimulation of the right cervical part of the vagus nerve has led to a drastically improved survival of subjects with induced Pulmonary Hypertension. This is further aided by treatment using pyridostigmine, a type of acetylcholine-based substance that helps increase the activity of the parasympathetic nervous system. This has been previously used to help improve left ventricular function, and is now being used to blunt the tone of the sympathetic nervous system, thus allowing the parasympathetic half to catch up and balance. The study is just touching the tip of the iceberg, since it still has not been translated to success in human samples.

Vagus Nerve and Alzheimer's Disease

Dementia is one of the most dreadful effects of aging, and nowhere is it more dreaded than in Alzheimer's disease. This illness continues to fascinate researchers, its roots being a cocktail of genetic and lifestyle-related concerns. It is also the source of some of the major medical breakthroughs of recent years. There was a time when Alzheimer's was a dead end, with no cure. Today, there are several options (albeit mostly experimental) that could pave the way for a definite cure. And of course, the vagus nerve has a huge role to play in exploring these possible cures -- though maybe not in the way you thought of at first.

As already mentioned, the vagus nerve is the highway that links the brain to the digestive system, what many researchers call the "gut-brain axis". The gut is home to a huge host of microorganisms, many of which are very important in regulating the response of the immune system. What isn't known to many is that this biome of organisms also has a huge role to play in one's mental health, so much that the term "second brain" has arisen in some circles. While some may consider this an exaggeration, it is true that the gut and the brain work with each other through the vagus nerve.

That is, the brain does not just control how the gut works, the gut also sends signals that affect the brain.

This becomes even more relevant to the topic at hand when we consider that an imbalance in the gut's host of microorganisms has been found to be among the roots of Alzheimer's. While age is still the primary risk factor in the onset of Alzheimer's, many other conditions have been found to be nearly as influential, among them obesity, issues with one's cardiovascular health (such as hypertension) and even depression. You would notice that these are also all conditions where the vagus nerve comes into play!

Recent research has focused on the treatment of Alzheimer's not from the brain, but from the gut and from the bundle of nerves that connect it to the brain. This research is given further impetus by the recent findings that Alzheimer's may partially be caused by infection from various types of viruses, in combination with a host of other factors. We already know that the vagus nerve has an important role to play in the regulation of the immune system, so this lends more credence to this emerging field of study.

Vagus Nerve and Memory Loss

But memory loss is not only exclusive for people suffering Alzheimer's. In fact, memory loss is very common, not only among the aging. For those who lack mental exercise, especially those with unhealthy diets and lifestyle, memory loss is a pretty common occurrence.

Again, the vagus nerve comes into play. The vagus nerve connects to the brain primarily through a relay network called the Nucleus Tractus Solitarius (NTS). This part of the brain connects the vagus nerve to the other parts that are related to memory and learning. Thus, stimulation of the vagus nerve can also lead to stimulation in these parts.

Memory improvement related to vagus nerve stimulation has not yet been thoroughly studied and conclusively proven in humans, but all signs thus point to this fact. For example, some studies in animal samples reported that those who underwent stimulation of the vagus nerve had better overall information retention and performance than those who did not. There had also been similar studies on human subjects with the same result, but a bigger sample set is needed for these studies to receive the stamp of scientific approval. It is to be noted that the changes noted were not immediate. Instead, they changed over time. This fact also calls for a longer study period to see just how far the memory-improving potential of the vagus nerve can go.

In all the examples so far, we have found how the vagus nerve, almost literally, has its fingers in all of the body's pies. It is one of those very important and yet very undermined parts of the body. Ignoring its importance can literally be a life or death situation.

Perhaps the most amazing is the fact that this bundle of nerves is so instrumental in fighting a host of so many illnesses that might appear too tough or too unusual to be dealt with by even the latest medications. It's all about understanding how the body works, and shifting the paradigm of treating these otherwise intangible illnesses to improving the restorative balance in the body.

Now that you have this information, how would you know if your vagus nerve is healthy? The next chapter deals with the specifics of vagus nerve health.

TAKEAWAYS:

- The vagus nerve's functions and connections allow it to influence a wide variety of diseases. These include:
    - Weight-related issues
    - Depression
    - Anxiety
    - Trauma
    - Epilepsy
    - Brain damage
    - Sleep issues

- Inflammation

- Pain

- Hypertension

- Alzheimer's Disease

- Memory Loss

- A healthy vagus nerve can prevent these issues from occurring, and can also help a person bounce back if they are already afflicted with such ailments.

CHAPTER 3: Is your Vagus Nerve healthy?

"The first wealth is health." -- Ralph Waldo Emerson

If you've never paid attention to your vagus nerve before, that's quite normal. In fact, unlike more famous vital organs in the body, the vagus nerve is very rarely heard of in normal conversations despite its importance. Those who might be hearing it for the first time would be forgiven to think of it as some pseudoscientific mumbo-jumbo -- in our world where nearly everything has one job and one job only, it seems inconceivable that something in our body aside from the brain (and perhaps the spinal cord) could be in charge of so many things at once.

However, this lack of knowledge about the vagus nerve can be quite debilitating. Put simply, there are lots of ill conditions that can occur due to a damaged or unstimulated vagus nerve. These issues are made apparent in the organs that the vagus nerve touches -- organs that are important not just in keeping our overall well-being, but also our vital processes.

Let's count the various injuries you may get from a damaged vagus nerve:

Starting with the nerve's attachment to the vocal cords, a damaged or inefficient vagus nerve can cause hoarseness and a strained feeling when talking. A voice that is unnaturally deep or hoarse, especially one that sets on without any actual damage to the pharynx or larynx can be a symptom of vagus nerve damage. You may also experience difficulty in swallowing, and the toning down of the gag reflex. The latter is important because it protects the body by automatically rejecting things that could choke us. A reduced gag reflex makes a person more susceptible to choking.

The vagus nerve is also connected to the ear, and plays a role in the brain's interpretation of sounds by carrying signals. Damage to this segment of the vagus nerve can result in partial or full hearing issues, ranging from the inability to distinguish sounds to deafness.

The organs inside the thoracic cavity are also innervated by the vagus nerve, so damage can also bring an increase in heart rate which can be harmful. This brings with it an increase in blood pressure, since the vagus nerve is responsible for the parasympathetic support to the cardiovascular system.

As for the esophagus, which is also connected to the brain through the vagus nerve, it can experience difficulty taking in food and drinks. The gut can also experience discomfort, or outright malfunction. Hyperacidity is a common symptom, which can damage the stomach's lining. The disruption of the established control mechanisms relating to gastric acid secretion can also lead to peptic ulcer due to the excessive secretion of peptic acid. This can also lead to other gastrointestinal issues such as dyspepsia.

When the part connected to the intestines are affected, this could cause problems in the process of peristalsis, the one responsible for moving food along for digestion and eventually absorption. Impaired peristalsis can cause constipation and other problems in the bowel movement. The urinary bladder is also touched by the vagus nerve, and damage can cause incontinence.

There are also several illnesses that can be caused or aggravated by a faulty vagus nerve, which sadly most people are not aware of. If you have one of the following, especially, read through this book as you will likely benefit from a healthier vagus nerve:

- Obesity or excess weight
- Depression
- Chronic fatigue
- Irritable Bowel symptom
- Irregular heartbeat, such as bradycardia (slowness of the heartbeat) and tachycardia (increased speed of the heartbeat)

- Rapid weight loss

- Peptic ulcer

- Chronic inflammation

- Gastroparesis

- Epilepsy

These is quite the varied list, and most of these diseases are caused by a list of factors. Because of the number of possible causes, most people don't even consider the importance of the vagus nerve in all this. But, together with the many ways one can rein in these diseases, taking care of the vagus nerve is also important.

Other, more generic symptoms of vagus nerve damage include the following:

Pain. This is the most common symptom, but also the one that tends to mask vagus nerve disorders the most -- simply due to the fact that pain can occur for a huge variety of reasons.

Pain due to vagus nerve is caused by the latter being pinched, often at the small exit through which it leaves the skull. While most other pains are sharp and stabbing, pain due to vagus nerve issues are mostly dull, and flat. It is also chronic, and while you can ease the pain through various means it is hard to completely get rid of it.

Cramps. Like pain, cramps are dreadfully common. Aside from the important organs we have mentioned, the vagus nerve is also connected to a few other muscles. While these muscles are not controlled by the vagus nerve per se, a malfunction in the nerve can also cause damage to the ability of the muscles to move. This includes cramps, which are different from those caused by a lack of electrolytes such as potassium and magnesium.

Fainting. As mentioned before, the vagus nerve also triggers fainting when overstimulated. When the nerve malfunctions, the same effect is achieved. Fainting per se is not life-threatening, but it does carry the risk of accidental injuries such as hitting your head or breaking a bone upon falling.

What causes vagus nerve issues?

Like most of the diseases enumerated earlier would suggest, certain lifestyle choices can greatly affect the vagus nerve' health. Here are a couple of the common activities that can degrade your vagus nerve's health. Note just how incredibly common these factors are in today's lifestyle, however. If you think that bingeing and boozing are destroying only very specific organs in your body, think again. That extra gummy bear might be leading to breathing difficulties in the future, thanks to the link between sugar, the vagus nerve, and the lungs!

Drinking. While occasional drinking isn't bad, chronic abuse of alcohol can greatly affect the nervous system as a whole, not just the vagus nerve. The more alcohol you take in, the more the nerves are damaged in a process called "alcoholic neuropathy". This causes severe problems throughout the whole body.

Sugar intake. Sugar is the main energy source of the body, and a healthy sugar intake (through complex carbohydrates) is also important. However, too much can cause diabetes, which can drastically change the chemistry of the nerve. This leads to such conditions as gastroparesis with symptoms including abdominal bloating, vomiting, and constipation. This happens when the stomach and the intestines are no longer able to properly push food through the digestive system.

Other causes of vagus nerve injury or malfunction are not related to the person's lifestyle, but rather are incidental to other issues:

Infections. Infections of the respiratory tract may redound to the vagus nerve. This can be pretty hard to pin down since symptoms can be indistinguishable between illnesses with infection at the root, and illnesses with the vagus nerve at the root. For example, both include runny nose, cough, and nasal congestion.

If these symptoms remain for long periods, however, it is likely that the vagus nerve is at fault, and it is also possible that a previous infection has caused it damage.

There are also infections whose symptoms include the inability to speak continuously, unusual tiredness of the throat, coughing, and the compulsion to clear the throat all the time.

Surgery complications. This isn't as common, but there are some times when operations done to the gut go wrong. A common surgery is the laparoscopic hemifundoplication, which is used as a treatment for one's gastric reflux. The damage happens when the surgery damages the vagus nerve connected to the stomach or the small intestine.

Repairing a damaged Vagus Nerve

Nerves are very fragile, which is why the most important bundles of nerves in our body are sheathed by tough layers of bone and cartilage. But the vagus nerve, alas, is pretty exposed -- exposed enough that when you press on your carotid arteries in the neck, you are essentially pressing on a part of your vagus nerve. Thus, the vagus nerve is far less protected from injury than other nerves.

For the most part, repair of the vagus nerve is symptomatic, meaning the symptoms are treated as they appear. Rarely, however, do such treatments actually go back to treating the vagus nerve itself. Fainting due to the overexcitability of the vagus nerve, for example, is treated by medication. Excessive or abnormal activity of the gastrointestinal tract is also treated by medicines, though some treatments have such side effects that most of them are reserved for more severe cases.

There is also the surgical alternative, though most only treat the symptoms. Patients with gastroparesis, for example, can go under the knife for stomach bypass or stomach staples.

Other symptoms of vagus nerve malfunction can be so subtle, however, that there are those who fail to detect them immediately and consequently don't take any steps to treat them.

Since it is currently impossible to isolate the specific part of the vagus nerve that is causing illnesses, there is no way to operate on it directly. The best option is a holistic approach that relies on stimulating the whole length of the nerve through the different points it is attached to. There are several ways of doing this, and it is even possible to address some issues directly through vagus nerve stimulation. We will be learning more about these techniques in the next chapter.

What to feed your Vagus Nerve

As we have mentioned, the best approach towards repairing and improving the vagus nerve is a holistic one. And there is nothing more holistic in approach than nourishing the body through the food we eat. Consider this section a rough guide on what food you should stock up on, in order to bring your vagus nerve back to tip-top shape. Of course, these are just general recommendations. If you think you have an injured vagus nerve, immediately go to a doctor who will give you specific advice on what to eat and what not to based on your individual circumstances.

The vagus nerve uses a type of chemical called acetylcholine as neurotransmitters. This acetylcholine transfers the information from the different organs the vagus nerve attaches to, towards the brain. The brain will then respond, sending acetylcholine down the vagus nerve towards the intended organ, mixed with other chemicals that would cause specific responses (such as anti-inflammatory ones).

Because of the importance of acetylcholine in the information transfer process between the brain and the organs, it is important to eat food that is known to help increase acetylcholine levels in the body. Here are the most common examples.

Egg yolks. Soft-boiled and raw eggs are great sources of choline. Cooking actually destroys the choline content, so if you are looking to use eggs as part of your vagus nerve diet, then it's best to keep it off the fire as much as possible.

Offal. Animal organs, such as kidneys and livers, are also great options for the improvement of one's acetylcholine levels. Pasture-fed sources are preferred, since these are less likely to contain harmful chemicals that can be absorbed by the body.

Lecithin granules. For the vegans, lecithin granules are perfect for building up the stock of acetylcholine in the body. These granules are usually made from soya, and sometimes from sunflower seeds. They can be added to different types of food and even drinks like smoothies.

Certain nutrients also help in the formation of acetylcholine, such as L-acetyl carnitine which can be found in meat. Various food sources such as squash and broccoli provide excellent sources of Vitamin B5, which helps in the creation of acetylcholine as well. If you like fish, you'd be happy to know that the methionine and lysine they provide can also be beneficial.

TAKEAWAYS:

- Like any other body part, the vagus nerve can be damaged. Damage can lead to a host of possibly debilitating symptoms, such as lifestyle diseases and chronic pain.

- This damage can be caused by lifestyle choices such as vices and improper diet, and also by injury caused by surgery and the like.

- However, the vagus nerve can be restored to health by proper stimulation and following a vagus-friendly diet.

CHAPTER 4: Jacking up the Vagus Nerve

"You have always to stimulate the senses." -- Henrik Fisker

Way back in 1934, a physicist found out that when the carotid sinus is pressed down, it produced a direct response in the circuit of the brain. This response cascaded into a difference in the person's heart rate and blood pressure. Such was science's entry into the field of vagus nerve stimulation that had been practiced without clear definition or direction for ages.

Only four years later, Bailey and Bremer noted that such stimulation caused changes in the reading of ECG results. In 1951, a different study showed that stimulation of the vagus nerve -- then isolated and severed -- had evoked changes in the thalamic regions of the brain. And finally, in 1985, there was the concrete observation that electrical stimulation from the vagal region inhbits some neural processes. This can change the electrical activity in the brain, and end seizures of an epileptic nature. This ushered in the era of using vagus nerve stimulation as a means of addressing illnesses.

Why stimulate the Vagus Nerve?

If the vagus nerve is so important, surely there is a way to make it better? If we can train the brain to be sharper, and our spinal cords to conduct instinctive movements faster, then maybe there's something we can also do for the vagus nerve. We know about muscles being exercised in order to strengthen them and improve their functioning. But how can constant stimulation improve the health of a nerve?

As an oversimplification, nerves are networks of neurons, "relays" that transfer signals (chemical impulses) from one part of the body to another. While neurons don't grow in size like muscles, it is possible to make the transfer of impulses faster and more efficient by "exercising" them through constant stimulation. This stimulation, when performed consistently over time, creates a physical change by improving the structure of the neurons, allowing them to be better at carrying signals. This is the principle behind such concepts as "muscle memory", which is in fact a certain set of neurons involved in the performance of an activity being conditioned to fire off faster and more efficiently.

The vagus nerve also benefits from the same concept. When the nerve is stimulated consistently, it becomes better at sending signals to and from the many organs attached to it. Thus, it improves several important functions of the body, from heart rate and respiratory rate to the digestive process.

Methods of Stimulation

Vagus nerve stimulation (which we'll call VNS, moving forward) can be classified into two. On one hand, we have the natural VNS methods, which are done without the aid of any electronic tools. We also have more modern methods that utilize implants and other devices that send electronic impulses directly stimulating the vagus nerve. In this chapter, we'll explore how both these methods work, and the benefits that each one has.

Natural Methods

Natural methods of stimulating the vagus nerve have been known to man since ancient times, but only recently have they been substantiated by scientific findings. Only recently had these same methods actually been connected to real-world physiological effects -- in the ancient times these practices were all about managing the flow of energy and creating a body that is one with the mind and spirit.

While natural methods have not been found to be as immediately effective or as well-targeted as their electronic counterparts, research has shown that there are concrete benefits to be had when stimulating the vagus nerve through these means.

Just like in electronic methods, natural methods can be done on demand and adjusted in "intensity" according to one's preference. However, since they don't target a specific part of the nerve, natural VNS methods give way to a "Goldilocks" principle wherein the person needs to find the perfect balance between stimulating and not stimulating the vagus nerve. For example, VNS may need to be done when one feels down or anxious, but too much stimulation can swing one's mood to the opposite direction and make him irritable and panicky. This cycle of ups and downs can alternate frequently, causing more issues than before. It is up to the user of natural VNS methods to find the middle ground.

Here are some of the most common ways to stimulate the vagus nerve naturally.

Humming. Since the vagus nerve passes through by the neck, attaching some of their ends to the vocal cords, it is possible to stimulate the nerve by simple humming a tune. In fact, humming has been found to be one of the easiest ways to influence the state of the nervous system.

When humming, do it with gusto -- you will know you are doing it right when you can feel the vibrations in your throat, and in your chest. When you have achieved a certain level of practice, you will also feel the vibrations reverberating in your head.

Immersion in cold. While most people shun the cold, it is actually essential in the stimulation of the vagus nerve and is as such instrumental in ensuring the nerve's health. In fact, multiple record-holder, Wim Hof attributes much of his incredible cold-related feats to an overall wellbeing that is primarily fueled by his cold-based training. He is not superhumanly resistant to cold, just like any human -- but his being accustomed to the cold has given him unusual levels of autoimmune development that allowed him to complete his feats.

A study suggests that as the body tries to adjust to the cold, the sympathetic nervous system slows down, and the parasympathetic system takes over. The sympathetic nervous system would be more familiar as the fight-or-flight mechanism, which is more active and is mediated by other nerves. The parasympathetic system (also nicknamed the rest-and-digest system) is triggered by ambient temperatures that are around 10 degrees Celsius.

Animal experiments also found out that sudden exposure to cold temperatures such as 4 degrees Celsius can greatly increase vagus nerve activation. This may be rooted to the fact that historically, creatures bathe in cold water in order to relax. Warm water was not easily available (in fact quite rare) even in the hotter regions. These conditions, before the advent of heating, seem to be the primary reason for the evolution of this response for the cold. Today, cold tubs are still popular in countries such as Japan, while many European countries neighboring the Arctic Circle also partake of cold ocean dips in special occasions.

If you want to try this out, but can't find the right conditions, taking a cold shower is a good place to start. You may pre-condition your body (and also your vagus nerve response) by dipping your face in cold water first. This will trigger the diver's reflex, which will be discussed in detail later.

Deep Breathing. Various deep breathing techniques can be used to influence the nervous system. The common denominator among these techniques is that the means of breathing employs the diaphragm, where the vagus nerve is attached. For most people, breathing is a matter of expanding the chest space through lifting the shoulders. This is an incorrect form of breathing, as it places undue stress on the upper chest, without actually working the muscle meant for breathing (the diaphragm). In correct deep breathing (and even regular breathing), the diaphragm moves and makes space for the lungs to draw in air. Physically, it looks like the stomach is bulging out, and the chest and shoulders stay in place.

The most effective deep breathing techniques for the stimulation of the vagus nerve involve slowing down the breath. The normal respiratory rate is at 10 to 14 breaths per minute, and deliberately slowing this down to about 5-7 breaths per minute can greatly increase stimulation in the vagus nerve.

One of the most common techniques not just for controlling the breath but also for managing stress is the "Box Breathing" method, so-called because of its technique of counting to 4. Basically, you breathe in for 4 seconds, hold the breath for 4 seconds, breathe out for 4 seconds, and hold it again for 4 seconds. Repeating the process has been known to calm the mind, especially in times of stress. It has also been known to reduce headaches and similar pain, which has been attributed to its ability to stimulate the vagus nerve.

Another technique one can use is prolonging the exhalation. A common counting system is breathing in for 5 seconds, and breathing out for 10 seconds. Aside from stimulating the vagus nerve, prolonging the exhalation helps ensure one uses up all the available oxygen upon inhalation.

A technique specific to the stimulation of the vagus nerve is the constriction of the back of the throat upon exhalation. This motion is similar to when one wishes to fog up a mirror or a piece of glass. The difference is that the air still passes through the nose instead of the mouth. This is a known yoga breathing technique, called *ujjayi pranayam*. There is a host of other yoga-related breathing techniques that you can try. Some of these techniques are downright unusual, but the common denominator is that they place a great strain on the diaphragm, therefore stimulating the vagus nerve attached to it.

If you feel like it, the breathing techniques involved with singing (particularly those songs with high notes and long verses) can also stimulate the vagus nerve. This is one of the driving forces behind the healing power accorded to meditative chanting. Singing hymns or repetitive chants can help activate the part of the vagus nerve that is at the back of the throat. A scientific study has found that for a group of 18 year-olds, singing can actually increase the Heart Rate Variability through VNS. Heart Rate Variability has been associated with better adaptation and resilience, along with relaxation. It also helps increase the efficiency of the body's rest-and-digest mechanism, an activity that is primarily overseen by the vagus nerve.

Later, in the second part of this book, you will be introduced further to the art and science behind breathing, and its place in the near-esoteric field of contemplative traditions. We will be breaking down the general ideas behind the concepts of meditation, mapping the science behind them, and from there building a new practice that you can use in your daily life.

Valsalva Maneuver. This may sound complicated, but it's actually just the act of exhaling (or, more correctly, attempting to exhale) when the airways are closed. This is a familiar technique for those who want to make their ears "pop" when boarding a plane, or when moving to a ground of different elevation. The maneuver is commonly used to equalize the air pressure in the ear, using the small ducts that connect the ears to the nose. However, the Valsalva Maneuver also helps increase the pressure inside the chest cavity, stimulating the vagus nerve from there.

The maneuver is done by simply keeping the mouth closed and pinching the nostrils shut, then trying to breathe out. Don't do this too rashly, as this may cause injury to the ear when forced. Test it out slowly at first until you can find the most comfortable intensity of exhaling.

Diving Reflex Stimulation. The "diving reflex" is essentially the body's ability to prepare for an underwater excursion. Such reflex changes the body's normal way of distributing oxygen, channeling the bulk of it to the brain and the heart, and reducing supply to the other organs and areas of the body. This is done in order to make the most of the oxygen stores and therefore prolong the ability to stay underwater without needing more oxygen. The vagus nerve is also involved in this process, and it is possible to do natural VNS by stimulating the diving reflex.

While diving reflex can be (weakly) stimulated by holding the breath, it can be better stimulated by contact with cold water.

Splash cold water on your face, especially on the space between the lips and the hairline. You can also simulate this by using ice cubes in a Ziplock bag. Couple the process with a moment of holding your breath, to trigger the redistribution of oxygen. If you don't feel like wetting your face, it is also possible to stimulate the diving reflex by dipping your tongue in lukewarm liquid. Hold the liquid in your mouth, and roll it around with your tongue, in order to evoke the reflex.

Making social connections. Weirdly enough, there have been studies that showed that the vagus nerve can be stimulated by positive emotions. In fact, it is possible to stimulate the vagus nerve by doing something that makes you feel happy and connected. This is different from simply feeling calm and at ease, since the latter (in the form of meditation) has been proven to be ineffective at natural VNS.

Another way to effectively stimulate the vagus nerve through making social connections is having a good laugh with a friend or family member. This is the reasoning behind the famous quote, "laughter is the best medicine". In fact, laughing has been proven in some clinical tests to be effective in natural VNS. One basic proof is the propensity of some people to faint while in a fit of laughter. This has been pointed out to be due to an overstimulation of the vagus nerve as well as other parts of the parasympathetic nervous system. Other means of overstimulating the vagus nerve can also lead to fainting. Another proof of the connection between laughter and the vagus nerve is the laughter elicited by electronic VNS in children with epilepsy.

Other studies seem to suggest that the *idea* of connection alone can increase the body's natural ability to stimulate the vagus nerve. A study involving a small group of people found that praying -- an act that elicits a feeling of connection to a higher deity or purpose -- helps increase vagus nerve activation. The group unanimously experienced an improved level of cardiovascular rhythms, and also had a drop in diastolic blood pressure. Other researchers pegged the VNS effect to the actual act of saying the prayer. Praying the rosary, for example, takes around 10 seconds for the reading of each cycle. When said orally, this effectively slows down the breathing pace of a person and regulates inhales to once every 10 seconds, thus producing the same VNS effect as measured breathing.

Probiotic intake. This is still an emerging field of study, but some research has suggested that the flora in the gut can have effects in the nervous system. Remember that the gut connects to the brain through the vagus nerve, so some researchers believe that good bacteria in the gut also translates to nourishment for the vagus.

There have been some animal studies that seem to prove this point, although in terms of scientific robustness they are still lacking. In one such study, mice which had been supplemented with a type of probiotic had experienced an improvement in the GABA receptors, among the many parts of the parasympathetic nervous system that is being regulated by the vagus nerve.

Physical Activity. There is more research to prove that a good dose of physical activity can greatly help improve the performance of the vagus nerve, stimulating it for better efficiency. Those into yoga, for example, will be happy to know that the mood improvements caused by the activity is greatly affected by the thalamic GABA levels increased when the vagus nerve is active.

Other forms of exercise help stimulate the flow of the gut part of the digestive tract, and this is caused by the concurrent stimulation of the vagus nerve connected to it. Like the probiotic angle, though, much research is still needed to support this claim, especially on human subjects.

Even if you don't like to move your body, you may still get good natural VNS by having a massage. Make sure to get a massage that reaches the neck area, as you need to target specific areas such as the carotid sinus. Research suggests that epileptics, or those who regularly get seizures, can get relief from this kind of VNS -- though it is not advisable to do it at home since overstimulation can result in fainting. The effectivity of such massage is so well-known in other regions that a neck massage is given to infants to stimulate their appetite (mediated by the vagus nerve). Finally, there are reflexology methods that purport to excite the vagus nerve as well, though these have been tested only in small experimental groups.

Diet Patterns. Since the vagus nerve is connected to the gut, there are ways to stimulate it directly from the changes we do to our diet patterns. For one, eating a diet high in seafood can give us EPA and DHA, omega-3 fatty acids that lowers the heart rate and heightens the heart rate variability. Heart rate variability is linked to the stimulation of the vagus nerve, and some scientists believe that this is a big reason why omega-3 fatty acids are so good for the body.

Zinc is also considered to be important to natural VNS through diet. In laboratory studies, zinc has been found to increase vagus nerve stimulation especially after a diet that is particularly deficient in it.

For those who are on a hard diet regimen, even fasting can help improve the health of the vagus nerve. Intermittent fasting has been shown to increase the heart rate variability in certain animals, and this is found to be a marker of vagus nerve stimulation.

As with many of the resources cited here, fasting still needs to be observed in bigger samples in order to establish its complete efficiency. One theory states that fasting mediates a reduction in a person's metabolism, in the same way that it mediates a change in a person's metabolic priorities in the diver reflex. This time around, the vagus nerve will detect a decline in the blood glucose levels, and a decrease in the mechanical and chemical stimuli coming from the digestive tract. This reduction has been found to increase the level of vagus nerve impulses from the liver to the brain, triggering the slowing of the body's metabolic rate. As always, check with your doctor when attempting to engage in any fasting regimen. As it stands, fasting can have more harmful effects than good one when done improperly, even if it does stimulate the vagus nerve.

Fiber, which is known as a very important component of a healthy gut, also has great effects on the vagus nerve as part of a diet. Studies suggest that fiber helps increase the occurrence of GLP-1, a satiating hormone that also has the effect of stimulating the vagus impulses to the brain.

On the other hand, it is also important to note that there are types of food that can serve to *inhibit* the vagus nerve instead of stimulating it. Carbohydrates, for example, increases the levels of insulin in the body. This insulin can compromise the function of the vagus nerve, which connects to the function of the liver. Capsaicin and ginger are also among the most potent ways of inhibiting the vagus nerve -- in fact, ginger's ability to stop vomiting and nausea is attributable to its ability to hinder the function of the vagus nerve.

Electronic Methods

Before we delve into the different methods of electronic vagus nerve stimulation, it's important to understand that these methods are not free from side effects. In fact, it is possible to feel these side-effects intermittently even while stimulation is not being applied.

These adverse effects, when present, can be felt in the organs that are connected to the vagus nerve. It is not that common, however, since as mentioned around 80% of the nerves in the vagus carry signals from the body to the brain, so only 20% are left with the ability to actually affect the body parts.

Different parts of the vagus nerve, when stimulated, can lead to different side effects. For example, left cervical VNS can cause changes in one's voice, as well as coughing. It can also affect the neck, causing pain. Dyspnea or shortness of breath is also a common occurrence. Right cervical VNS, on the other hand, has been known to produce bradycardia or the slowing of the beating of the heart. In extreme cases, especially when stimulation (or the device applying it) is misapplied, it is also known to cause asystole or the lack of contraction in the ventricle of the heart. This is a form of cardiac arrest, and is deadly.

Despite these possible adverse effects, direct electronic VNS is a very potent cure for various conditions as we will shortly see. The most important thing to remember is, like any other medical treatment, to have it done by a licensed medical practitioner well-skilled in the process. This way, electronic VNS can immensely improve one's quality of life.

Is it safe for me?

The adverse effects mentioned here can all be controlled by changing the parameters of the device used for stimulation. Generally, tolerance to side effects build up as exposure to the stimulation is prolonged. There are no known recurring adverse reactions which would endanger a VNS patient, and even children and pregnant women have been treated successfully by the technique. Its combination with medication has also been well-studied, and unless indicated by your doctor should have no contraindications.

The only limitation is that a person carrying a VNS implant could not undergo such radiation-based procedures as MRI, and shortwave, microwave, or ultrasound diathermy. Diagnostic ultrasound is still permissible. The implant is also not affected by common radiation-emitting appliances such as metal detectors, microwaves, and cellphones.

Left Cervical VNS

In the left cervical VNS, stimulation is done by the implantation of a "pulse generator device". This is commercially available, and its "installation" is a quick outpatient procedure done under general anesthesia.

The generator is placed just under the skin, in the left upper chest. It has an electrode that is attached directly to the vagus nerve via another incision made in the left neck section. The electrode and the generator is connected via a lead wire. Since it is a relatively simple procedure, there aren't many things that could go wrong. The installation of the pulse generator is generally safe.

The generator itself is programmed by a handheld computer, interfaced with the device through a programming wand. The wand is passed over the skin where the device is implanted. There are various parameters that can be controlled, which the doctor can program. These parameters (intensity, charge, pulse width and frequency, etc.) are all optimized to deal with the specific illness the stimulation is treating.

These generators typically run continuously, and the only way to turn them off is to run a magnet over them. This is only temporary, though -- only the programming wand can turn it on or off completely. The battery life can change depending on the parameters set, and when spent can be easily replaced.

Right Cervical VNS

This is the technique used in order to help reduce seizures in animal models. It has also been looked into for the treatment of depression, but human tests on the matter is still inconclusive.

Like in left cervical stimulation, a device is also implanted in the body. However, an additional system has been developed for VNS stimulation leading to the treatment of heart failure. This device is implanted in the patient's right chest wall, and is connected via a cuff to the right cervical vagus nerve. This cuff is meant to activate specific efferent fibers of the vagus nerve, in order to fix the cardiac rhythm. The device has a stimulator which responds directly to the heart rate, shutting off when the heart goes past the threshold for bradycardia.

Studies have found that stimulation of the right cervical vagus nerve is not only safe, but also effective for the treatment of heart problems. In Israel, a similar system has been designed specifically to counter any possible VNS-related side effects. This device, in contrast, only activates the afferent fibers. This right cervical VNS device has been used in conjunction with the left cervical VNS-based treatment to improve the status of patients without causing any untoward side effects.

Transcutaneous Vagus Nerve Stimulation

There are also devices that can stimulate the vagus nerve at different locations through a person's skin.

For example, the outer ear carries the vagus nerve's auricular branch, and this nerve exclusively services some areas of the ear. One such area is the cymba conchae, which can be stimulated by applying an electrical stimulus. The stimulus can be felt by the person, but is still below the pain threshold. Such a stimulation can produce activity in the brain that is similar to direct stimulation in the left cervical vagus nerve. Hence, this can also be used to help treat epilepsy and some other types of pain.

Aside from being much less invasive than direct stimulation, another advantage of transcutaneous VNS is that it can be applied by the patient himself. What may be an issue, though, is the fact that there are no universally accepted clinical processes on the application of transcutaneous VNS. The manufacturer of the stimulation device (currently the only one approved for clinical use) says that stimulation sessions should last at least an hour, up to 4 times a day. The literature behind this recommendation is still unclear, but the device's effects are substantiated. Pilot studies have also been done on the product's efficiency for depression epilepsy, pain, and some other complications. While the results are yet to be verified by bigger studies, there is already a universal consensus on the product's safety.

A different device has been approved for use for the treatment of migraine, cluster headache, and headache due to the overuse of certain medicines. The device, called "gammaCore", is a handheld device with two flat surfaces that can be placed over the neck where the pulse is. The device then sends an electrical signal which lasts for about 90 seconds. The intensity is controlled by the patient, and the device may be used on demand when headaches come, or throughout the day to prevent headaches. While there is some literature supporting the effectivity of these devices, it still needs larger trials for further proof. Unfortunately, there are no trials yet to prove that the same device is useful for epilepsy and depression, two other areas where VNS should be helpful.

TAKEAWAYS

- A huge number of techniques can be used to stimulate activity in the vagus nerve. Stimulation is important to make the vagus healthier, hence improving its function and improving the overall health of the body.

- Vagus stimulation may be natural or electronic:

  - Natural methods can be done through variations of engaging the lungs (humming, deep breathing, singing, etc.) or engaging the reflexes of the nervous system (cold immersion, Valsalva method, etc.). It is also possible to stimulate the vagus nerve through psychological means such as fostering a healthy social life.

- ○ Electronic stimulation is done by implants, targeting different parts of the vagus nerve. There are also implants that are done at skin level, which are less complicated and have a broader (less specialized) range of stimulation.

PART 2:

The Vagus Nerve in your Daily Life

Thus far we have discussed the scientific points of the vagus nerve along with the many options one has for stimulating it.

But what we have so far is a disparate set of information, things that are illuminating but not immediately practicable in daily life. It's like trying to learn how to train in martial arts by knowing only the descriptions and mechanics of various punches and kicks, and the materials one needs to have to train, but not really applying them in one's everyday living.

In this unit of the book, we will try to combine everything we have learned so far in order to distill a functioning "vagus nerve training manual", one that you can do even in the midst of your hectic schedule. After all, one of the main reasons why the vagus nerve weakens in the span of the modern lifestyle is because so few of us actually have time to train it. Here, we will try to remedy this by creating a set of vagus-stimulating activities that can fit in no matter what backdrop of activities you may have in your daily life.

CHAPTER 5: Vagus Nerve and Meditation: An Ancient Combination for Modern Life

"Meditation is not following any system; it is not constant repetition and imitation. Meditation is not concentration." -- Jiddu Krishnamurti

Thanks to popular media, the image is all-too-familiar to the modern generation. A lone man, well-advanced in his years, sits alone on a mountaintop, still and silent, deep in meditation. When he stands up to do his chores, he does it slowly and rhythmically, without any hurry. Approach this old man and you would be amazed at his wealth of wisdom, and his flawless recall. You would be even more amazed when you find out that this man must be nearly twice as old as he looks! If ever you make the regrettable decision of being mean to this man, you would also feel that his strength and coordination has hardly declined since his youthful days.

This image seems all too magical, a mere invention by people who glorify the ways of the old, who romanticize the quiet life of the mountain sage. Myth and legend are rife with such figures of impossible feats, but the fact that they no longer exist in the modern day makes their possibility patently questionable. And yet, in every story is an iota of truth. What if there *were* such people, with such traits? Sure, stories of their feats had been exaggerated, but where did people get the idea that a life spent alone and in meditation could unlock near-supernatural powers within an individual?

With the discovery of the vagus nerve and all its potential, we may have found the answer.

The Art of Contemplative Traditions

Earlier in this book, we have discussed that there are ancient methods that have been known to increase the vagus nerve stimulation. We have also discussed the many separate ways through which vagus nerve stimulation can be attained, either naturally or electronically.

Short of actually having a vagus nerve implant (which can only be had if one actually has an illness treatable by such a device), then what we need for daily life is a holistic approach that can serve to uplift our general wellbeing as much as it uplifts the vagus nerve. This is why for this chapter, we will look into one of the most time-honored "rituals" that can be embedded in one's life, as a thorough approach to VNS. We are looking at contemplation -- a very broad array of practices with the common goal of improving one's overall health. In study after study, science has also proven that these are among the best ways to improve vagus nerve health.

The Treasure Trove of Contemplation

Contemplation takes different forms. Some may be introduced to it in the modern takes on meditation. Others may be more focused on the schools of knowledge passed down in yoga or tai chi. All of these acts have ancient roots, and all of these have been found to have immensely beneficial effects on the physical, mental, and cognitive well-being of a person.

However, there haven't been many studies actually elaborating on how these practices achieve their efficiency. A 2018 research, however, posits that all of these practices have one thing in common, and it is this one thing that makes them so efficient -- in all of them, breathing is carefully controlled and guided. Yoga, tai chi, and simple meditation are not just a series of postures, they teach a form of regulated breathing that helps stimulate the vagus nerve. We have already gone into slight detail about how to help stimulate and tone the vagus nerve through simple exercises earlier, but this time we will look at these methods as something that can be applied to all corners of daily life.

For the purpose of this chapter, we will be referring to the collection of similar contemplative actions as "Contemplative Traditions" or CT. These CTs are usually done in order to help one achieve a more "balanced" life (though balance may be a word whose meaning slightly differs depending on the specific practice). They are also aimed (and proven effective) at changing one's state of mind. They appear in several forms, from praying to meditating. Let's dive into the understate treasure trove of these traditions with a brief history.

Meditation is a set of traditions that come from the Asian region, usually rooted in the Hindu or Buddhist belief system. There are different types of meditation from each country of origin. For example, China birthed the origin of Zen meditation, while India was the cradle of transcendental meditation and vipassana. There is also the loving-kindness meditation of Tibet. These have all seen popular resurgence, with various studies supporting their efficiency.

According to the 2018 study, these meditative acts can be generally classified into two: Focused Attention (FA) and Open Monitoring (OM). The former trains the person to focus on a single point, object, or action, and to shift the focus back to the object being meditated on should a rogue thought arise. Open Monitoring, on the other hand trains the person to spread his attention thinly across multiple stimuli, those things happening around and within him, so that no single item has his rapt attention. Some traditions blend from one meditative practice into another, with OM being seen as more advanced models of meditation than FA.

A broader classification of meditative processes, found in a 2015 study, is based on the emphasis in techniques. This resulted in a three-way classification: attentional, constructive, and deconstructive. Both FA and OM are then found under the banner of attentional meditation. Constructive meditation is aimed at internal improvement and the spread of such improvement to others. An example is loving-kindness meditation. Then, there is the type of meditation that removes the barriers of everything from habits to perceptions, from thoughts to behavior. This is exemplified by most forms of mindfulness meditation. Note that we are solely referring here to mindfulness as a meditative practice, and not as a state that is achieved after indulging in such practice. As a state, mindfulness can be the target of any other meditative techniques, particularly those of FA and OM.

Then again, there is a whole different subgroup of the meditative practice dedicated to the synergy of the movements of the mind and body. These include all forms of meditation that include stances and complex movements, along with those that include muscle relaxation techniques.

These classifications are important because the effects of vagus nerve stimulation are more pronounced in some categories than in others, simply due to the fact that there is a different set of instructions given for these meditative practices. But research has found that all of these practices have at least some type of effect in the various domains of wellbeing. Here are a few:

Improved cardiopulmonary functioning. Various CTs have been shown to decrease risk factors concerning a person's cardiorespiratory health. As much can be found from various meta-analysis studies that compared independent research on various CTs. Some practices, though, like qi gong, have not yet been efficiently studied due to a lack of long-term trials.

Anti-Inflammatory effects. Many CTs have records of improving immunological improvements, centering on anti-inflammatory effects. These effects have been quantified in the reduction of pro-inflammatory markers in the body, along with a reduction in the cytokines that ignite inflammation.

General physical improvements. This is where it gets pretty interesting, as many CTs have been found to improve bodily factors as diverse as bone density, physical balance, and overall strength. These changes also help alleviate pain, and this includes not just muscular pain but also illnesses such as migraine and osteoarthritis. Stress reduction has also been found to be a direct effect of these physical improvements. These effects are, in fact so strong that they are comparable to the medication used for chronic pain.

Decrease in stress-related issues. We have mentioned that stress-reduction is a common result of these CTs, and naturally the reduction of symptoms of illnesses related to stress would follow. These include symptoms of psychopathological illnesses such as PTSD, anxiety, and depression.

Improved cognitive control. Some studies have also shown that CTs can enhance the way the brain handles memory and other executive functions. These are the functions that rely on high-level mental processes, such as arithmetic and logic. These improvements can act as a remedy for many memory and logic issues related to age-related brain decline. These improvements are especially pronounced in mindfulness-type meditation. Just like in physical improvements, these mental improvements can be so pronounced that it is possible to induce them simply by short bursts of CT interventions. These effects could snowball after prolonged exposure to such practices.

Improved attention span. Most practitioners of CTs would attribute their improved ability to concentrate on everyday tasks to their constant practice at keeping their attention during the meditative stage. While the idea that "willpower is a muscle" still remains debatable, research lends credence to it thanks to studies showing a specialization on attention and focus for those who practice CTs.

When we say "attention span" here, we're not just talking about the ability to stay focused on one task. Different CTs offer different advantages according to their nature. For example, Focused Attention (FA) CTs increase one's ability to sustain attention on a narrow field for extended periods, while those who practice Open Monitoring (OM) CTs have the ability to jump from one mental task to another without muddling the ideas that come to mind. Both of these types show just about the same level of enhanced mental performance overall.

Improved creativity. Creativity is not something that is easily measured, so studies on the matter are limited to easily observable traits such as verbal creativity. Various CT researches have proven that practitioners have increased levels of creativity over time, coupled with an increase in the overall cognition ability. This latter metric consists of various thinking exercises such as convergent and divergent thinking. Practitioners are also better able to distinguish the many things happening around them in daily life, pointing towards a better level of awareness, which in turn helps fuel their creativity.

When we look at all these benefits from CTs, it is easy to draw the line between the observed improvements and the vagus nerve. All these improvements touch areas of the body, both physically and mentally, that are directly connected to the vagus nerve's many functions. Thus comes the proof that these meditative practices, discovered and practiced since ancient times, holistically improve the body by engaging the vagus nerve.

What makes these CTs so effective?

These CTs have their own unique traits, which we need to look into so that we can discern just what makes them so effective. After all, not everyone has the time to study yoga or tai chi, and not everyone has a place they can go to for Zen meditation. We need to determine what principles and techniques are at play, which make these practices so effective.

In 2011, a study on mindfulness meditation has revealed a formula-like set of activities that are common to most CTs. These include attention and affect training, the adjustment of "metacognitive recognition" (simply put, being aware of what one is aware of), awareness of the body (including its states and processes), physical activity, and the use of various breathing techniques. Let's take a look at these factors, and how each would affect the vagus nerve.

Attention and Affect Training. In CTs, the focus on attention isn't very clear cut. Several traditions train one to focus on an external object, while others teach one to focus on internal processes such as breathing. Still, some would push for a focus on abstract concepts such as thought, and the very idea of thought. Then, there are some CTs (such as the first incarnations of Zen meditation) where one isn't taught to focus on anything at all.

As stated earlier, the type of attention training would greatly affect the cognitive improvements one may reap. Some are able to focus on a task even better, while some are able to multitask without much distraction. Thus, it would be better to understand attention training as something that is more focused on control rather than on a specific result.

Affect training, on the other hand, is focused on training a person to handle one's emotions and moods. This means being aware of what one perceives to be negative feelings and ideas, and turning them into something that is useful or at least manageable. This is a more abstract equivalent of exposure therapy, wherein one is exposed to negative stimuli in the hopes of giving him time and means to process it so it makes less of an impact.

Most CT practitioners are instructed to "alter" their mental state by diffusing the intensity of the negative thought or emotion. Most practices would teach their students to consider that these are all just fleeting sensations, therefore allowing the student to detach himself from the idea that is observed. The detachment that then results protects the practitioner from forming any more of such ideas.

In effect, attention and affect training covers two important parts of the mind: the cognitive and the psycho-emotional parts. As discussed previously, these parts are both also affected by the vagus nerve. This is why VNS has become important areas of research in the battle against Alzheimer's (cognitive) and depression (psycho-emotional). Furthermore, it has been studied that a better grip on both one's conscious and subconscious thought processes is an effective way to prevent the onset of extreme stress. Reduced stress then allows the vagus nerve to start its own healing regimen, leading to better immune function and heart health.

Adjusting one's metacognitive recognition. CTs are well-known for their overarching concepts of oneness, unity in everything. This is also evident (perhaps not surprisingly) in how the common denominators of these CTs present a unified front. Case in point is metacognitive recognition, which is a direct effect of the techniques used in attention and affect training.

Metacognition is better put as "thinking about thinking". Therefore, adjusting metacognition is changing the way one thinks about thinking. At first blush, this is an idea that is meant to twist the vagus nerve and the brain into confusion, but in practice, it can be fairly straightforward -- just focus on changing the way your mind processes information.

The brain is very good at recognizing patterns, perhaps so much that most of the stimuli we encounter everyday have a "default" response as they go through a certain route in the brain.

These instincts and impulses then shape our reality. While these may be put to good use, such as in committing certain actions to "muscle memory" (really a practiced pathway from the brain to the muscles) for faster retrieval, sometimes these also lead us to spirals of negativity. This is why many CTs advocate "thought monitoring" in order to teach us how to deconstruct thoughts and how we process them, moving away from default responses and preconceptions to carve new processing routes and possibly new outcomes.

At face value, this seems to be the root of how creativity is improved for those who practice CTs. When practiced, it helps a person gain better control over how he processes information, getting rid of irrelevant ones and providing a fresh perspective on the relevant ones (potentially allowing for new and novel uses).

Such a process helps improve the overall health of the vagus nerve in a way that is different from most of what we have discussed so far. We have touched upon the idea of "muscle memory", which is in fact just an improvement on the pathways that send signals from the brain to specific areas of the body, in order to trigger a specific set of responses. The benefits of metacognitive adjustment to the vagus nerve runs in the same vein. Looking at old stimuli in a new light will transfer the information to new areas of the brain, passing through those areas of memory and emotion that are also served by the vagus nerve. When these stimuli elicit new responses, a different part of the vagus nerve may be activated in order to serve the flow of new information.

Nerves are "exercised" through the process of myelinization. Myelin is that substance that sheaths the nerve fibers around the axons, allowing for efficient transfer of signals from one nerve to another. The healthier the myelin sheath is, the faster the travel of information from one end of a neural network towards the other end is.

Myelinization is triggered by using the same network over and over again -- this is why we are able to pull off instinctive reactions to stimuli more quickly than newly-acquired responses. But if we are able to pull back from such preset networks to explore other possibilities, then other parts of the vagus nerve can also undergo the process of myelinization, therefore strengthening the whole network. In contrast, disuse of specific parts of the network, whether it is in the vagus nerve or in other parts of the body, would make the myelin sheath weak an inefficient at transmitting information.

Awareness of the body. Certain CTs instruct practitioners to be aware of the body and its different states, often focusing on the tension in the muscles or sensations in the skin. Still others would instruct practitioners to focus on what their "gut" tells them (though very few actually recognize the existence of the gut as a "second brain" as discussed earlier).

In keeping with the theme of oneness, this bodily awareness is also central to the whole affective process discussed before. Body awareness teaches the CT practitioner to treat the body as a separate entity, a vessel that contains the self, but that is not completely the self. This encourages a culture of interoception (this time connected to the idea of metacognitive recognition), and teaches one to be keener in understanding what it is the body feels. Studies have expressed the fruits of this practice as an increase in tactile acuity, and a resulting increase in the parts of the brain that process the signals being sent by the body. These, in turn, can produce vivid effects on the emotional and cognitive levels.

This benefits the vagus nerve in the same way that metacognitive recognition does, allowing the brain to intensively engage new sections and possibly new pathways through the vagus nerve.

Physical activity. Many would point to the physical activity practiced in different CTs to be the primary factor in their effectiveness as harbingers of wellbeing. However, this is just one side of the coin, as we have demonstrated with the effects mentioned above. Still, the physical benefits reaped from CTs that recommend activity stand out on their own, even while directly interplaying with the other benefits discussed above.

It is also to be considered that some CTs do not advocate any specific type of physical activity at all, such as the sitting meditation of later Zen meditation schools and the prayer meditation practiced in some religions. Still, these have not been found to be inferior to the more physical CTs. This points to the fact that overall benefits can be gained simply from the internal processes of CTs, especially the concomitant vagus nerve stimulation.

Like in benefits to mental acuity, the various improvements in physical ability would depend on the specific contemplative tradition that is being practiced. For example, some schools of yoga place special emphasis on flexibility and on aerobic endurance. Tai chi, on the other hand, focuses on balance and posture. There are some studies positing that aside from the physical benefits these actions provide, they also help increase a person's cognitive health since physical control is directly mediated by the brain. There have also been some studies that say these actions can improve working memory, though the results are still debatable.

One curious point here is the fact that there is no direct evidence to point to the physical activity involved in CTs as a direct source of the mood-enhancing effects that are attributed to such practices. A review in 2009 mentioned that even increasing the physical components of CTs don't correlate to actually increasing their mood-enhancing factors. This points to the fact that there are more important factors at play for those who wish to gain mental clarity from meditative practices. Also, it is noticeable that of all the CTs studied by various experts, only a select few actually have exercises significant enough to produce significant boosts in the physical makeup of a person.

Cardiovascular health, which is among the primary benefits of physical activity, is directly connected to the health of the vagus nerve. In the previous unity, we have already mentioned how cardiovascular health is inextricably linked to the vagus nerve, going so far as to determine a cardiovascular metric as a manifestation of the vagus nerve's health. While drowned out as a primary candidate for vagus nerve stimulation at least in the field of meditative practice, it is also interesting to note that activities that trigger increased cardiovascular excitement have their fair share in boosting the vagus nerve's health.

Before moving on to the next common denominator in CTs, let's pause for a moment to synthesize the different factors we have learned so far. Theorists have put forward separate ideas that serve as models determining the effectivity of CTs. Some of them have focused on the primacy of the CTs' focus on executive functions of the brain, pointing to these as the most useful aspect of developing the person. Others point to the synergy of mind and body, pointing to the superiority of mind-body movements coupled with exercises that focus on attention. There are researchers who encapsulate CTs as a form of "meditative movement". However, such researches may be faulted for relegating movement to simply motor coordination, almost completely omitting the aerobic benefits (however mild) that some CTs have.

TAKEAWAYS

- Contemplative Traditions hit the sweet spot on many different bodily issues. Incidentally, these same issues are also those touched upon by the vagus nerve, serving as the first hint towards their interconnectedness.

- There are various types of CTs, but they all have similar basic sets of rules. These rules then serve as the primary drivers of their effectiveness.

- When done properly, these rules complement each other to produce a snowball of health effects.

CHAPTER 6: Breathing, the Foundation of Life

"Breathing in, I am aware of my heart. Breathing out, I smile to my heart and know that my heart still functions normally. I feel grateful for my heart." -- Thich Nhat Hanh

We have saved the breathing discipline aspect of CTs for a separate chapter to highlight just how vital it is to the overall idea of meditative practice -- and also to highlight how it is the foundation of all that is vagus-stimulating in the practices we have highlighted so far.

You've already read how diaphragmatic breathing is a key to stimulating the vagus nerve, and you've also seen different techniques to induce such stimulation in a jiffy. But since we're going for a holistic system rather than a one-off technique, let's discuss breathing a little in-depth, and in the context of these contemplative traditions.

On top of the theories discussed in the preceding chapter, two researches (Gard, in 2014; Wayne and Kaptchuk, in 2008) have also put forward a breath-centric model to explain the ability of these CTs to induce wellbeing. The researches went on to describe the breathing patterns used in traditions studied to be "slow, deep, and diaphragmatic" -- just the exact combination needed for vagus nerve stimulation.

The breathing techniques are undoubtedly meant to slow down the respiratory cycle. For many traditions, the exhalations are much longer than the inhalations. The "focus" of breathing becomes the abdomen -- that is, the person should be conscious not of the air entering his nose and going down his chest cavity, but of the same air filling the lungs and the lungs pushing out the stomach. This is the "natural" breath, the type one can see in children and infants before they are conditioned by stress to take quick, shallow breaths. The only exceptions in CTs are some techniques that specifically use faster respiratory cycles, such as in a few yoga techniques. But these are in the minority. Some meditative traditions aim to make a synergy between these slower breaths and the movement of the body. In essence, the pace of the breathing is the foundation -- the rest of the body will follow.

Breathing, such a basic act, has been described in many a scientific literature -- but rarely in such a way that describes its role in the contemplative traditions. This is despite hard evidence showing that breathing is the single most effective factor in attaining the purported benefits of these meditative practices.

So let's take a look at what sparse evidence there is to see breathing in action. According to a 2008 study by Danucalov, there is an increased metabolism and oxygen absorption in the body during breathing exercises prescribed by yoga traditions (pranayamas). This is a surprising finding, since meditation usually invokes the idea of resting and relaxing.

Such breathing exercises studied included breathing in and holding the breath, then extending the exhalation as far as one can go. A 2009 study of the same set of pranayamas found that despite increased internal activity, there has been a registered drop in blood pressure for the subjects studied. There was also an accompanying reduction in heart rate. A more focused study on Sudarshan Kriya Yoga, also done in 2009, found a general activation of the parasympathetic nervous system to induce a rest-and-digest state, wresting control from the sympathetic nervous system.

Breathing by any other name

Some studies have also taken the breathing exercises out of the context of CTs and attempted to manipulate the regular breathing states of test subjects to see if they can influence the dials of the autonomic nervous system. A study, for example, quantifying the difference between normal (unconscious) breathing and diaphragmatic breathing found that the subjects had a reduced heart rate and a higher insulin content in the blood when they consciously breathed. Another study in 2001 found that a hypoxiated individual can oxygenate the blood faster by breathing in and out slowly rather than by regular breathing. These studies were duplicated in 2015, with the same results.

While there are a few researches with conflicting data, the bulk of the scientific facts currently available contend that conscious, diaphragmatic breathing -- the type espoused in a vast majority of CTs -- can on their own increase a person's wellbeing. The other techniques found in CTs are meant to build upon this vital bedrock, exploiting and multiplying its benefits.

Breathing Science: Linking it to the Vagus Nerve

Now, how exactly does the vagus nerve play a role in all these, especially in breathing? We know that the vagus nerve is stimulated by breathing, but where does it go from there?

To answer this, we need to look into a model called the Neurovisceral Integration Model. In this model, it is hypothesized that there is a bi-directional relationship between the autonomic functions of the nervous system and the cortices of the brain. The model posits a system called the "Central Autonomic Network", whose purpose it is to modulate the rest of the body's autonomic functions. The parts of the nervous system involved in this network then interface with the endocrine system (that collection of organs which are involved in secreting hormones to affect the other functions of the body). This interface is done through -- guess what -- the vagus nerve.

But the Neurovisceral Integration Model also suggests that the communication works both ways, and that the rest of the body, through the endocrine glands, can also communicate with the autonomic network through the vagus nerve. In effect, this creates a loop. The brain sends signals to the body, the body responds and sends feedback to the brain, which it then uses when sending another set of signals out. Other sequences are also possible, such as when the brain focuses on its executive functions and signals the body to relax. Thus, a healthy and stimulated vagus nerve is both an indicator and a means of creating a sturdy link between a well-responding nervous system and a well-relaxed body.

To simplify things, breathing and CTs help stimulate and improve the overall wellbeing of the vagus nerve. This wellbeing, in turn, serves as the platform on which the body builds a working network of feedback and balance mechanisms. When done long enough, it is possible for these breathing practices and CTs to produce structural improvements in the autonomic network.

The Neurovisceral Integration Model also plays to the strengths of meditative practices. The stress-busting effects of mindfulness, for example, can be explained in terms of adjustments in the influences of external stimuli on the network. For example, an exaggerated response to a trigger may be reconsidered (and therefore be treated less as a stressor) by either reappraisal (top-down approach, stemming from the executive functions and moving down to the visceral level) or continued exposure (bottom-up approach, where visceral-level stimuli affect the executive function).

Boiling it all down

As we've mentioned, the reason we're going through all this trouble is so we could identify the most important factors that make contemplative traditions so much of a success, in an attempt to bring these lofty practices down to a level that can be called on at any time in our hectic lifestyle. Most contemplative traditions are steeped in philosophy, which can be a good avenue for a different type of learning and practice. But for those who just need to maintain vagus nerve health for daily wellbeing, something much more basic would suffice. Think of it as Cliff's Notes for contemplative practices. They can work on their own, but now that you know the science behind them, you can expound and make modifications whenever you wish.

Let's first take a look at the things we have distilled from our discourse into CTs, so far:

- Breathing is the central component of meditative practice, and the main stimulant for the vagus nerve. Slow breathing and slow exhalation is the most prevalent form in contemplative traditions.

- Awareness of the body, the mind, and the surroundings plays an important role in stimulating the vagus nerve by letting signals flow to various areas of the brain and body, in a way that makes new neural pathways or improves old ones.

- Physical activity is not a must, but it can also help build new neural pathways through the vagus nerve.

From these, we can now construct a new and more potent vagus nerve stimulation regimen.

TAKEAWAYS:

- Breathing is not just one of the most essential of bodily processes. Done right, breathing can also serve as the primary stimulant of the vagus nerve.

- Scientific studies have found that breathing not only helps relax the body, it also helps manage the various stimuli that enter our senses.

CHAPTER 7: Breath-Centric Stimulation

"To build may have to be the slow and laborious task of years. To destroy can be the thoughtless act of a single day." -- Winston Churchill

Contemplative traditions are very multi-modal, and they're not to blame. After all, if one seeks to attain purity in life, he would do well to occupy his time with useful stuff. Most meditative practices are made to occupy a man's time just enough so that he cannot be idle.

But this cannot apply to our daily lives. Today, we live in a world of perpetual avalanche. Everything just falls down endlessly, and to take time to breathe means to fall several steps behind. There have been very famous meditative techniques that invite a person to pause for at least a minute to "breathe in the present". But soon, that present becomes the past, and (with due respect to meditative schools that espouse the idea of the "eternal present") the time taken to meditate could just lead to further stress as one regrets the time he could have spent doing something.

This is not to disparage the contemplative arts. They are still highly recommended, and they can be truly life-changing experiences. But it would be difficult for the everyday salaryman -- the man most stressed, the man whose vagus nerve is most likely frayed beyond recognition -- to step away from the hamster wheel even for a moment. Thus the drive to create something that can be integrated seamlessly wherever one is, whenever one needs it.

And this has resulted in something *so* simple indeed that it would be harder not to use it in daily life.

"Bullet Time" Breathing

Here is a meditative technique where you do not need to stop whatever you're doing. You do have to slow down, to keep your breath in check, but at least you can balance your productivity with your vagal health.

It goes like this:

- Several times throughout the day -- as often as you need it, depending on your stress levels -- take one, big breath. This should be a breath that originates from the diaphragm, not from the chest cavity. Feel your diaphragm push your stomach out, and draw in as big a breath as possible. Then, exhale with force. This will serve as a mental cue of what happens next.

- For as long as you can afterwards, breathe in and out slowly. It is not necessary to count the seconds as you breathe in and out. Just be aware of the same sensation of air filling your lungs and of your diaphragm being pushed out. You don't need to take your mind off your task at hand, either. Just relish the air going in and out, as slow as is comfortable. Note that your "slow" might still be fast at first, but constant practice will allow you to lengthen your breaths and lower your respiratory rate even further.

- As you do this, slow down in whatever task you are doing. The idea is to match the pace of your task to the pace of your breathing. If you are typing on your keyboard, for example, slow down just enough so that your fingers don't feel out of rhythm with your breath. If you are walking, slow down enough just so you could feel each breath. Here, you are making your breath the foundation of the moment -- and everything else afterwards is just an accessory to it. The slowing of your task is meant to provide as little distraction as possible to your breathing rhythm, since you are trying to maintain this for as long as possible.

- If you notice that you are breathing your normal pace again, that's okay -- you don't have to spend too much conscious effort trying to maintain your slow breathing. At first you won't last very long, but this will change with constant practice. It's even possible that constant practice will allow you to turn slow, diaphragmatic breathing into a normal habit! It is hence advisable that each time you notice that you're breathing fast again, to begin the process anew.

- If remembering to take that one big breath before you start slowing down is difficult, try setting an alarm or using different cues in your surroundings to remind you to take it slow. If your schedule permits it, you can also set something to guide your breathing as you enter this phase. A metronome, for example, could greatly help (make sure to set it on a slow beat). Other natural sounds such as the hum of the AC or the ticking of the wall clock may also be used as rough guides for breathing (just make sure not to follow the clock by the second -- the longer the interval the better).

Just like the iconic "bullet time" sequences in movies, this technique of slowing down carries with it just enough weight to let you see what may otherwise be imperceptible things (attention and affect), give you time to notice new things about old stuff (metacognitive recognition), allow you to observe your own motions by slowing down (bodily awareness, mixed with physical activity), all while exciting your vagus nerve through slow, diaphragmatic breathing.

Too Simple? Not Quite

There are those who would decry this type of technique as too simplistic, and not completely taking advantage of the many good things that true-blue meditation has to offer. And yet, it still ticks all the scientific checkboxes.

One may find it unusual that no special emphasis is given to maintaining the breath for a set period of time. In fact, the instructions are kind of vague when they talk about how long you should maintain the breathing pattern, and how slow it should be. But according to research of existing contemplative traditions, simply using the breath as an attentional focus will immediately yield changes in the respiratory rate. That is, a person who focuses on his breath will unconsciously slow it down. Deeper breaths automatically follow. The idea with the first conscious, deep breath is to set a template for the body to follow in its automated slowing down, while also conditioning the mind to be aware of the mechanics of deep breathing.

Another interesting fact about respiration-based vagus nerve stimulation is the fact that it is a bilateral process. This is as opposed to other vagus nerve stimulation systems, especially the electronic ones. Of all the vital functions in the body, breathing is the only one we have conscious control of, so any change in breathing pace would have a more profound effect on the whole body than any other conscious action. These effects can be classified into either direct or indirect functions:

Direct Function. Among the direct functions of "bullet time" breathing, mediated by the stimulated vagus nerve is the lowering of one's heart rate and blood pressure. This is due to the cardiorespiratory coupling through the vagus nerve previously discussed. This process is the one that famously reins in the sympathetic nervous system, and activates the anti-inflammatory pathways (with which, again, the vagus nerve is involved). This then helps reduce stress levels, and over time can increase cognitive control through the Central Autonomic Network.

Indirect function. After "bullet time" breathing has affected the nervous system, this relaxed nervous system would then send respiratory signals back to the lungs, this time signifying a low-threat scenario. Thus, the way one breathes is now being affected. The expansion of one's abdominal cavity to accommodate the lungs is more pronounced. This cycles back quickly to affect cardiopulmonary patterns. As the loop goes on, the anti-inflammatory effects of the parasympathetic nervous system are engaged, along with an increased cognitive control.

It is also to be remembered that this better breathing pattern causes an increase in the oxygen levels of the blood, thus providing more fuel for the brain and other organs. This also helps further sharpen the cognitive improvements charted from vagus nerve stimulation.

While the indirect route takes time to take hold, it is not any less important. In fact, the indirect functions are being investigated as the initiator of long-term improvements in vagal tone.

In contrast, other forms of stimulation would only result in one-dimensional improvements, and most of these are hardly sustainable. With "bullet time" breathing, however, it is possible to achieve all the long-term effects attributed to a healthy vagus nerve without needing to take precious time off your daily tasks. Such a routine can be carried out with minimal effort and can be squeezed into whatever you're doing. Whether you're indoors working on a project or outdoors making your way past the commute, you can take your sweet "bullet time" to get your life and your vagus nerve back in order.

TAKEAWAYS:

- Slowing down your breathing, and doing so in a mindful manner, is enough to get your daily vagus nerve exercise without taking time off work. The exercise filters all the best practices of contemplative traditions into a holistic yet unobtrusive process.

- "Bullet time" breathing exercises can be done as follows:

  ○ Take a deep diaphragmatic breath, and exhale with force.

  ○ Take all succeeding breaths as slowly as comfortably possible.

  ○ Try to maintain this breathing pattern. Slow down your movements by being synchronous with your breath.

CHAPTER 8: For that Quick Pick-Me-Up

"I don't fear death because I don't fear anything I don't understand. When I start to think about it, I order a massage and it goes away." -- Hedy Lamarr

There are times, though, when you might want a more sensory experience to wake up your vagus nerve. These may come at times when you quickly need energy, or when you need to perk up for an upcoming activity. As mentioned in the first part of the book, massage and reflexology can help stimulate the vagus nerve. But if you're all by yourself, you can also stimulate your vagus nerve through a massage.

In this chapter, we'll put together all we know about vagus nerve structure in order to create a routine massage you can use for a quick pick-me-up.

Step 1. Start from your collarbone. Put your fingertips in that fleshy part where your collarbone meets your neck, and massage upwards. You may increase the sensation by going for one side first, then the other.

Step 2. Place your fingers behind your earlobes, in that soft part right under the skull. Massage in a circular motion.

Step 3. From there, move your fingers downward. The target this time is the back of the neck, on either side. Massage the area slowly downwards.

Couple this massage routine with slow, diaphragmatic breathing, and you will feel relaxed. And yet, you will be energized enough to gain additional focus on the task at hand.

To cap it all off, you also need to mind your posture when performing your tasks. Man evolved an upright form not just in order to stand out from its fellow animals, but also to alleviate pressure in its internal organs — this includes nerves, such as the vagus.

A poor posture restricts the flow of information in the vagus nerve. This is especially prevalent when adopting a posture where the head juts forward or backward, thus putting pressure on the vagus nerve that goes out from the base of the skull. This can disrupt the nerve's functions, the most common effect of which is poor digestion and difficulty in breathing.

Today's gadget-dominated lifestyle has increased the risk of incorrect posture more than ever, that for some people their default posture is already broken. If you are among these, it might be good to visit a physical therapist for corrective therapy.

TAKEAWAYS:

- A "vagus nerve massage" is a good way to get your vagus nerve perked up immediately for those times when you need to perform harder.

- Proper posture is also important in maintaining vagus nerve health.

PART 3:

The Future of Vagus Nerve Stimulation

Thus far, we have gone through the current state of knowledge and technology with regards to vagus nerve stimulation, though we have ventured into some theoretical discussions along the way. This time around, let's focus on the theory and emerging fields of research in the topic of vagus nerve stimulation. What exactly does the future hold?

CHAPTER 9: The Vagus Nerve Versus the World

"I never think of the future - it comes soon enough." -- Albert Einstein

Aside from the vagus nerve, there is perhaps one other discovery on the nervous system that has shocked the scientific community, allowing research to strike off in new dimensions that could have unprecedented fruits. This is the fact that the brain is not a permanent blob of neurons -- that is, it can be molded and reprogrammed almost at will.

Now, we have the magical vagus nerve, and scientists are quick to make the link between the nerve and the brain's plasticity. Now, new avenues of research are looking into the vagus nerve as a means of engaging this ability of the brain to reshape itself.

This idea is the foremost being brought to bear on the topic of neurological diseases. Preliminary research has found that the brain's plasticity can be triggered by the norepinephrine and acetylcholine bursts that the vagus nerve excites. Thus, VNS is being looked at as a safer and more effective means of healing the brain.

120

It's a Plastic World

The concept of plasticity is straightforward enough. When the environment changes, the brain has the ability to change its "form", pretty much like a plastic can take on different shapes depending on the mold. Such plasticity can be called on for all kinds of tasks, from something as mundane as learning something new to something as staggering as recovering after a comatose or a debilitating injury. There had been reports of people waking up after years of coma, after their brains rewired themselves to go around the damaged portions. This is, so far, the upper limit of brain plasticity that we have registered.

Currently, the concept of plasticity is also being applied to treat all kinds of disorders. For one, there's the case of amputees who experience phantom limbs and phantom pain. Certain therapeutic methods are used to help rewire the brain's maladaptive behavior, helping it "realize" that the part of the body a small section of it is serving has been severed. This reorganization of the brain is usually induced through a variety of means, but in the future it is hoped that vagus nerve stimulation will play a part in making the process faster.

The same idea has been thought of as a possible research point in the treatment of tinnitus, which like phantom limbs perceives that something is there (this time, sound) when in reality there is none. As of the time of this writing, research is still lacking the correct neural map that the vagus nerve needs to stimulate in order for the renormalization process to proceed.

The Vagus Nerve as a Helping Hand

According to some studies, the existence of transmission in the brain can either promote or inhibit its ability to create new neural pathways. By "transmission", we mean the presence of chemicals that are associated with mental activity, such as norepinephrine and acetylcholine -- the two neuromodulatory transmission agents induced by the vagus nerve.

The lack of such transmission agents has been found to reduce the brain's ability to reorganize itself as needed by its surroundings. This comes up as a problem not only during moments of neurological damage, but also during times when the brain needs to adapt to external stimuli (such as when we are learning something new). Studies have observed the loss of plasticity in such wide-ranging mental functions as seeing and movement.

On the other hand, the presence of transmission agents in the brain have been found to enhance its plasticity. Some experiments have tried directly injecting acetylcholine to the brain during certain activities, and the brain responded accordingly by making minuscule adjustments in the spot.

Over time, this resulted in better performance in test tasks. Like in inhibition, such effects have been observed in wide ranging functions, which have also included seeing and movement. It has also been found that when the brain already has previous experience performing the tasks being boosted thanks to the presence of neurological transmission agents, such experience can be brought to bear in helping the brain strengthen its newfound connections.

The same principles have also been studied in brain activities that do not demand immediate action, such as in learning new concepts and theories. Research has found that the same level of plasticity can be leveraged during the acquisition phase, or that part where the brain collects all the necessary information to learn something new.

Oddly enough, the effect seems to fade during the consolidation phase, or when the brain actually tries to store all the gathered bits of information. From this, we can infer that the presence of neurological transmitters could increase one's ability to gather new information and store it as temporary memories (the amygdala, where short-term knowledge is stored, has been shown to be especially active in this stage) but whether or not the same information can be recalled after some time depends on other factors entirely.

This is very exciting news, as we are now seeing the birth of vagus nerve stimulation as applied in learning and training.

While the above-mentioned example has included the technique of directly injecting neurotransmitters into the brain as a sort of supplement, such an approach is impractical in everyday life. The only other alternative is to use the nervous system itself to stimulate the production of the same chemicals. And -- you guessed it right -- this can be done through stimulation of the vagus nerve.

Your Brain, the SSD

In the world of technology, we have created storage devices that have increasingly faster read/write speeds. Solid State Drives (SSDs) for example have unprecedented access speeds, allowing us to store and retrieve data faster than ever before. Wouldn't it be nice if our brains could also attain greater access speeds, so we can store stuff better and faster? But this has been found to be almost possible now, thanks to an outcrop of the research above. Simply put, there has also been evidence that plasticity can be used as a driving force to "control" memory.

The vagus nerve is also responsible for relaying information from the peripheral nervous system to the central nervous system. It relays two types of data -- one is "good" data, which soothes the brain (the feeling of satiety, or the feeling of relaxation, for example) and the other one is "bad" data (the feeling of stress, or the feeling of inflammation). These bits of information are then used by the central nervous system to help build memories on.

Because of this, an arm of research has also been thrust towards the idea of controlling memory through nerve relays and the transmission of this peripheral data. The extent is not yet completely known, but the vagus nerve has been showing participation in a lot of neuromodulatory tasks involved in the induction of plasticity in the brain. Electrical stimulation has already been shown to increase the activity of plasticity-driving chemicals in the vagus nerve. In the same experiments, a different link was also established -- without the presence of enough neuromodulators in the brain, even electronic stimulation would not have much of an effect in changing the behavior of the central nervous system through the vagus nerve. This points to the primacy of more natural methods of stimulation that rely on a healthy vagus nerve, not just one that electronically beats it into submission. The "bullet time" breathing technique described above makes for a good candidate for natural interventions to create the environment for such a healthy vagus nerve.

The Vagus Nerve as a Neurosurgeon

We have already touched upon the possible use of vagus nerve stimulation as a means of curing such conditions as tinnitus and phantom limbs, but if we are to push the boundaries of its ability to control plasticity then we might as well apply them to much more serious diseases. Among them is the dreaded stroke.

Stroke can be so debilitating that around 85% of stroke patients suffer from some sort of impairment in the upper limbs. Strokes cause a blockage in the blood flow to the brain, thus leading to cell death in the motor cortex. This death interferes with other motor-related circuitries, therefore leading to impairments in coordination and motor function.

As of this moment, there are no clear ways to reverse the effects of stroke. The only hope is to do therapy in order to regain some of the lost movement, and to hope that the brain heals itself. Now that the ability of the vagus nerve to induce plasticity has been uncovered, researchers are now looking at VNS coupled with motor therapy in order to help rewire the brain and regain complete motor function. Earlier research (from as far back as 2001) had revealed that the brain can reorganize its motor cortex much faster when VNS is used together with therapy. Tare are no known studies yet done on stroke patients, but this just remains part of the unexplored potentials of vagus nerve.

What other debilitating neurological issues can you think of? Some diseases likely to come to mind would be Parkinson's and spinal cord injury. And yes, both of these can also be helped by the vagus nerve's ability to stimulate neuroplasticity. The idea comes directly from the nerve's ability to help in the therapeutic treatment of stroke, and though the pathology of the three conditions are far apart from each other, the future ability to perform targeted plastic therapy can greatly promote healing by engaging undamaged circuitry in the brain. Brain damage due to trauma may also be helped by the same technique.

Aside from curing physical ailments, plasticity may also be invoked to help those with a cognitive disorder. These include those suffering from anxiety, stress, PTSD, and the other issues we have discussed earlier. This can also be extended to cover such issues as drug addiction, bipolar disorder, schizophrenia, and ADHD. While these are all issues with widely differing pathological origins, they all have a common denominator — they all include some form of cognitive issue, coupled with maladaptive plasticity. The entry of VNS in the field of possible treatments for these issues mark another landmark, and that is the attempt to address the underlying pathological issues of these illnesses. For a long time, treatment for these have also been symptomatic and their complex origins are undermanaged. Now, we have a way to try and fix how the brain works by fixing it through its own terms. As a plus, VNS might just be that flexible treatment platform which could address the special need for less regimented strategies for these health issues.

Note that this is not something of a magical cure to otherwise debilitating diseases. The idea of inducing neuroplasticity does not mean the brain can immediately repair itself. It is a mere boost to the usual process of therapy and recovery. Yes, it has the potential to drastically cut the time needed for recuperation, but there is still a huge gap between existing research and actual results.

One of the more pressing research questions is, just how much vagus nerve stimulation is needed to induce plasticity. The word is not yet final, but what we have is pretty encouraging.

Just add a pinch of VNS

According to recent findings, the frequency that's needed in vagus nerve stimulation for the process to be helpful in inducing plasticity is lower than the currently approved frequencies used in vagus nerve stimulating machines. As we have discussed in earlier, some of these machines deliver frequencies that can be felt by the user. For the most part, the sensation is tolerable, and one can easily grow into it. However, it would still be better if the frequency is left under the radar.

Studies have found that the current needed to induce plasticity via VNS is about 100 times less than that which is advocated in current protocols. This is foreseen to have fewer side effects. This same level of current has also been tested for the improvement of motor control through plasticity, and it is also the current used to help stroke victims during experiments of VNS use for recovery.

This, however, does not discount the possibility that the current recommended level of intensity for other applications of VNS (such as epilepsy and depression, where one needs a 30 Hertz pulse every 5 minutes, each one lasting for 30 seconds) would remain. There are other benefits from increased stimulation, such as the increase of neurotransmitters which could help drive other benefits not achievable with lower stimulation levels. Then, there is also the difference in the natures of plasticity-targeting VNS and existing commercial electronic VNS. For the latter, stimulation becomes more effective after a prolonged exposure. Meaning the issue being treated becomes more responsive to the pulses. For plasticity, however, the effect lasts only for as long as the stimulation is applied. This means VNS will have to be done at the moment it is needed, as the effect wears off immediately after.

As of the time of writing, researchers are yet to be able to map the exact frequencies needed to induce specific effects. When such a mapping is done, it would be much easier to customize frequencies as needed for electronic stimulation.

On Demand Sensory Relief

We've already discussed how the vagus nerve helps mediate pain and inflammation, and how stimulation can help eliminate these issues. Moving on from this knowledge, we can also look into the possibility of the vagus nerve as a means of controlling sensory perception and curing sensory dysfunction.

ain may be an important indicator of danger to limb, but it is at the core a type of sensory dysfunction. Vagus nerve stimulation may be just the perfect tool to remove the use of potentially addictive oral medication from the pain treatment equation, and it is also an ideal tool to help "normalize" sensations received elsewhere in the body. Sensory dysfunctions can be anywhere from irritating to debilitating (from phantom pain and itches to phantom limbs) and the vagus nerve can help reduce the intensity of dysfunctions so they don't drown out normal sensory input.

The Vagus Nerve as a Health Barometer

By now, you should be able to link a huge variety of health issues to the vagus nerve. You might mean it as a tongue-in-cheek idea, but you're not really far from the truth — at least according to a concept paper completed and published in 2018. It turns out that the vagus nerve is indeed THAT tied to overall health that its activity can be used as a barometer of wellbeing, sans the presence of communicable diseases.

This runs through the whole gamut of the Global Burden of Diseases (GBD, and yes that is an actual term), from cardiovascular diseases, to pulmonary issues, to cancer. Despite a disparity in their origins, it is possible to distill their roots to reveal a set of lifestyle factors (think stress, diet, and vice). The paper leverages known neuro-immunology data to use the vagus nerve as a predictor of the onset of such diseases.

According to the paper, the vagus nerve's connection to the front of the brain makes it related to an individual's conscious decision to make unhealthy lifestyle choices (which ultimately leads to diseases in the GBD). High activity of the vagus nerve, read through a high HRV, has been found to predict a reduced risk of GBD illnesses. The same level of activity has also been seen to increase one's hopes of bouncing back when beset with such a disease.

The paper also shows high hopes that this understanding of the vagus nerve can help alleviate not just the symptoms but also the roots of these GBDs, and advocates additional study on populations that have these illnesses.

The Vagus Nerve as an Antiseptic

Sepsis, stemming from bacterial infection of the body, is a huge medical problem. The issue arises for a multitude of reasons, and while medicine has made incredible headway in addressing septic issues, it still remains a multi-billion dollar thorn on the side of modern medical practice. But, maybe, advances in vagus nerve research can help stop the scourge once and for all.

We already know that the vagus nerve has mechanisms that allow for the control of inflammation, allowing the body's parasympathetic nervous system to soothe symptoms. But this is just the top of the iceberg. Research has showed that the same mechanism has pushed back the progress of sepsis in a number of patients, by regulating the release of the body's natural defenses against such infections. The increase in acetylcholine triggered by the activity of the vagus nerve has allowed the body to launch a chemical counteroffensive against the invading bacteria, stopping the spread of infection even without the use of pharmaceuticals.

These findings are especially important in the case of neonatal sepsis, or the type of infection that causes a significant mortality rate among newborns. These infants have underdeveloped immune system, making the very susceptible targets for infection. At the same time, they do not have built-in tolerance for a wide variety of pharmaceuticals, so a drug-free way to control infection is much sought after. The only blocker right now is the development of a device or technique that will allow newborns to have enough VNS to push back infection without using implants.

The research that made these findings had another, curious result. They found that the same vagus nerve stimulation needed to reduce infection has also been the same stimulation needed to arrest various breathing problems associated with preterm infants! When understood further, VNS techniques could knock a huge chunk off infant mortality rates. Later on, the same studies could be extrapolated for adults, too. And in a way, there have been similar attempts...

Breathing In Vagus Nerve Benefits

We've discovered how the vagus nerve can trigger the brain to release self-healing (essentially, self-transforming) chemicals, but that's not the only major organ that can benefit from the vagus nerve's wonders.

Recently, VNS has also been looked into for the treatment of lung injury — specifically one induced by ventilators during hospital confinement, whose pressure could rupture the alveoli (the little grape-like air sacs in the lungs that allow oxygen to transfer to the bloodstream). These same injuries are also often accompanied by sepsis, resulting in pulmonary inflammation.

Being one of the main organs affected by the vagus nerve, the lungs benefit greatly from the vagus nerve's ability to reduce inflammation. By regulating this inflammatory response, the nerve also makes way for the healing process that results in a significantly faster recovery rate. The process, however, has only been proven effective in tandem with pharmaceutical interventions.

Of course, if the luug can benefit from its connection to the vagus nerve, then the gut — significantly more connected to the vagus nerve as a sort of second brain — should also benefit. This is proven by some research, which found that gut and lunch injuries can be treated together in a "two birds with one stone" approach. There have been some studies that show how most septic issues in lung injuries are caused by bacteria breaking through the intestinal walls and getting into the lungs. Such movement is arrested by the vagus nerve's ability to regulate the permeability of the gut. This regulation of gut permeability has a role to play as well in the prevention of other gut-related diseases, though this field still needs more study.

"Will Vagus Stimulation Work For Me?"

As the vagus nerve moves from being an object of interest to becoming an actual point of cure, people will start answering whether or not vagus nerve stimulation will be the right treatment platform for them. In the recent past, the simple answer was "we'll never know until we try." However, thanks to a recent slew of research, scientists have uncovered a possible way to assess the future effects of VNS on a person.

We've already covered the idea of Heart Rate Variability (HRV) and how it can be gleaned from one's ECG results. But the vagus nerve's primary connection is to the brain, so it's only conceivable that there are external telltale signs pointing to the vagus nerve if we observe the brain.

According to a study concluded just this May 2019. measuring the reactivity of the patient's EEG results could point to whether or not he will be responsive to VNS treatment. These EEG scans are taken during the routine preoperative stages. By observing the dynamics and activity of the EEG results of a set of patients, the researchers were able to create a predictive formula that discerns one's possible VNS response by anywhere from 80% to 90% accuracy. While the model needs to be subjected to more rigorous tests by the scientific community, this could usher in a new era for VNS treatment by letting doctors determine the people most likely to benefit from these revolutionary treatment techniques. Remember that, at least for more serious cases of depression and epilepsy where one needs to be implanted with a VNS device, there are still possible complications that may arise from the operating process despite the relative safety of the stimulations themselves. By choosing likely candidates for success from the get-go, it is possible to determine whether the chances of success are well worth the risk of going under the knife. Think of it as a skin test of a whole new level.

TAKEAWAYS:

- Future avenues of vagus nerve research open up new possibilities. In the future, it may be possible to foretell one's health status and predisposition to diseases through the vagus nerve. It might also be possible to cure erstwhile incurable conditions of the brain and nervous system. For healthy individuals, future techniques and studies may be used to improve brain performance drastically.

- It will also be possible to foretell just how effective vagus nerve treatment on a person will be, thus better assessing risks versus potential rewards.

CHAPTER 10: New Devices for New Techniques

"With the new day comes new strength and new thoughts." -- Eleanor Roosevelt

Back in the day, the idea of operating on a person was a horrid experience. You just need to Google for images of operations back in the 1800s to fully appreciate the horror. Stil, the idea of manipulating the human body from the inside in order to promote health was a novel concept with an amazing breadth of applications, so physicians embraced the process.

Of course, progress soon followed, and techniques have improved drastically. Nowadays, it is possible — common, even — to go under the knife in the morning and walk out of the hospital in time for lunch. New techniques merited the creation of new devices, and this is something that can be seen as well for these developments in vagus nerve stimulation. After all, the vagus nerve represents the modern equivalent of "manipulating from the inside" in order to promote health.

True to Form

One of the most common issues with current vagus nerve stimulation implants is the latter's inherent inflexibility. The electrodes that interface with the vagus nerve are rigid, whereas the nerve itself is not. The problem is also present in other neuromodulating implants, where the electrodes may rub against the nerve and cause damage during movement. There have been reports of such implants causing damage to the axons of the nerves, the part where the transmission of neural signals from one nerve fiber to another happens. Manufacturing electrodes that fit the vagus nerve precisely would also be difficult and impractical, since everyone's measure is completely different.

To get around this, a team of Chinese researchers have created a type of electrode that takes inspiration from the climbing ability of vines and some other plants. Using a type of "memory metal", which changes shape under certain conditions (usually heat or electricity), the researchers have been able to create a type of electrode that conforms to the individual shape of the person's vagus nerve. This means doctors can now create implants that do not pose the threat of mechanical damage to the person's nerves. It would still take some time before this process is refined, and mass-produced. However, this would represent a huge leap in electronic VNS.

Perhaps an advancement that would hit the market sooner would be the new microelectrodes that researchers hope can deliver better therapeutic value by fine-tuning which parts of the vagus nerve will be targeted. These microelectrodes have the potential to stimulate just a very specific part of the nerve, connected to a specific function. This is expected to reduce side effects as much as possible.

In 2018, a team of researchers have created a different use for microelectrodes. The current model of VNS using electrodes is by sticking the electrodes into the nerve itself, and delivering electronic impulses from there. This necessitates a fairly complicated operation procedure. Instead of this, the team created a type of "wraparound system" using microwires that hug the vagus nerve instead of going through it. Fixed in place then insulated, this technique achieves a small footprint and allows for good contact even during the patient's movement. Perhaps more importantly, the technique can be potentially applied on awake patients without the need for a general anesthesia. Thus, in the future, it would indeed be possible to have a microwire planted into your vagus nerve in the morning, and you can still make it to your favorite place for lunch.

Mapping the Vagus Nerve

Another challenge, directly related to VNS (especially if we're talking about microelectrodes) is the inherent complexity of the vagus nerve. While we have a rough idea of which part activates what, we still do not have enough data on the vagus nerve's internal workings.

A Stanford study back in 2018 seeks to remedy this, and in a big way. Earlier in this book, we described how cytokines help relay neural signals from one part of the vagus nerve to another. The Stanford researchers used these cytokines as a type of marker that would enable them to map the way neural signals in the vagus nerve work. This opens up a way for future researchers to map the way signals weave their way through the vagus nerve, and (coupled with a knowledge of how these signals are transmitted chemically through cytokines) to potentially intervene with these signals to drive a certain outcome.

TAKEAWAYS:

- Using futuristic shape metals, microelectrodes, and more could usher in an era of safer and more effective vagus nerve stimulation.

- In the same vein, efforts to map the transmissions of the vagus nerve can also greatly improve the effect of stimulations.

CHAPTER 11: Paying It Forward

"Who will take responsibility for raising the next generation?" -- Ruth Bader Ginsburg

Let's face it — most of the issues we have today (health-wise, at least) stem from our upbringing and our adjustment to the modern world. Everything from stress to illness is a by-product of our fast-changing world, a world that we are forced to live in before we actually come to know how to *properly* do so.

This is the same issue with many of the issues that touch the vagus nerve and its complex network. Everything from poor diet and vice, to bad posture, to shallow and hasty breathing, is an adaptation to the world — and pretty ineffective ones, too. Unless we put a stop to the factors that inhibit the proper functioning of the vagus nerve (and thus the whole body), the effects will snowball to the next generation. And this generation will have a much more difficult time as the effects of vagus nerve impairment is felt with greater force.

An essential part of growing up

Nowhere are the myriad functions of the vagus nerve more pronounced than in infancy, when the body is still developing the advanced functions that will come into full play as an adult. During infancy, the vagus nerve has been found to be associated not just with physical development, but also with socioemotional development.

In experiments, the vagus nerve of term infants were stimulated through massage therapy. The researchers have found that this produces gastric motility, which helped drive weight gain and therefore growth. Aside from massage therapy, however, the researchers have found a different way to stimulate infantile vagus nerves — close proximity to and positive interactions with their mothers. In contrast, low vagal activity has been recorded for those infants whose mothers are depressed, angry, or anxious. Infants later found out to be autistc also showed low vagus nerve stimulation even when in a synchronous activity with their mothers.

This caused the researchers to look into the vagus nerve's involvement in the emotional growth of a child. It has been found that the more active the vagus nerve is, the more mature the overall structure of the autonomic nervous system is. Furthermore, when the vagus nerve activity is compared across a sample of term and preterm infants, it has been found that those with a higher vagal activity in infancy ended up to have better social skills, mental processing abilities, and motor skills. In contrast, those with low vagal stimulation during infancy were more likely to have less competence in the aforementioned factors. These have been followed up to school age, and the results are mostly constant. What's even more surprising is that using vagus nerve activity as a predictor for these factors ended up a much more accurate measure than other birth metrics such as birth weight, family health history, and even the economic status of the child's family. The researchers went one step further and tried to measure the vagus nerve activity of infants in the 36 to 40-month gestation period (done by observing a pattern of respiration and heartbeat in the fetuses) and found that the same conclusion holds.

VNS Should Start in Youth

It's one thing to try and raise a child to understand the importance of the vagus nerve and its effects to body, and another to try and insulate him from the vagus-tearing factors that persist in the outside world. How much one tries to do either or both will depend on his parenting style. One might want to teach a child how to do "bullet time" breathing when stressed, and another might increase the child's intake of vagus nerve-friendly food.

But while what happens at home is up to the parents, what happens in hospitals should be regulated by doctors and scientific evidence. And all evidence points to the fact that the vagus nerve plays a very important role in the wellbeing of a child, so much that its assessment and stimulation should be standard process in the battery of medical tests and procedures a child undergoes.

The aforementioned study looked at the case of preterm infants and those with low vagal stimulation, and found that techniques such as kangaroo care (close contact between mother and child) and massage therapy are effective and non-intrusive means of stimulating the vagus nerve. When these interventions were done, preterm infants showed a rapid maturation of vagal activity. Other aspect of infant life were also affected. The study noted that those who received kangaroo care ended up having longer hours of quiet, peaceful sleep and better alertness during waking hours. The periods of restless, active sleep were also reduced. The same study, done in Korea, also noted that infants receiving tactile and kinesthetic massage had increased levels of vagus nerve activation compared to those who did not receive such an intervention. Upon follow up studies, the researchers found the massage group to have grown more alert, more attentive, and more organized than their peers. They also had less instances of being underweight — back in 2007, a study detailing the effect of vagus nerve stimulation in infants noted that even without consuming more calories, infants who underwent VNS had better weight gain than others.

To drive home the importance of vagus nerve stimulation as a part of child development, a correlation was also drawn by the study between speech development and vagal activity.

According to records, a child that has better vagal activity is more likely to exhibit a wide array of positive emotions. This child is also more likely to vocalize earlier and more actively than his peers. They were also found to have better temperament than others.

It is also to be noted that the success of vagal stimulation on infants depends greatly on the vagal tone of the mothers as well. A mother who has a low vagal tone is very likely to pass the same to her child during face-to-face interactions. Children born of mothers who are depressed, for example, have been found to have elevated levels of cortisol — the stress hormone that activates the sympathetic nervous system as a response to perceived threats or pressure in the environment. And note that this happens at a time when the child should have no concept yet of stress! The elevated cortisol levels are also combined with a decreased level of dopamine and serotonin. Since the vagus is also responsible for innervating the facial nerve, one can easily see how an infant reflects a mother's blank facial expression.

To the Land Before Birth

Perhaps even more shocking than these findings is the fact that researchers have found a link between a mother's low vagus nerve stimulation before her child's birth, and a similarly low vagus nerve activation of the child upon birth.

Specifically, those expectant mothers who have a high level of anxiety or anger during the second trimester of pregnancy appear to pass on their vagal tones to their children. This has been attributed to the tendency of infants to mimic the biochemical profiles of their mother while in development. The infants are consequently born with low serotonin and dopamine levels, and high epinephrine and cortisol levels. In effect, they are born anxious, depressed, and angry!

The idea that one could "fix" these issues after birth is also met with difficulty. According to a separate research, the vagus nerve shows the most active myelinization rates during the first nine months of life — inside the mother's womb. While the child is still unborn, the myelinization process already "bakes" preset neural pathways in his vagus nerve, therefore preconditioning himm to certain responses. If these myelinated pathways are the wrong ones, you would have a child that is already preconditioned to have low vagal activity.

The message is clear. For us adults, all these talk about vagus nerve stimulation could either give us a better shot at wellbeing, or could maintain that wellbeing. But for children, vagus nerve stimulation could literally define the rest of their lives. Sure, there are individual differences, and the vagus nerve may not be a 100% accurate system of predicting a child's development. But to argue that, we would be entering into a theory that spans a vast multitude of systems. Some of these systems can be completely out of our control, such as the social order and physical environment in which we choose to raise our children. But that does not take away the fact that the vagus nerve *is* among the many systems at play, and at least this one can be controlled.

One could continue arguing that a child's future will in fact be determined by how we choose to raise them, but consider this. Children with subpar vagus nerve activity are often found to be more difficult to handle during the formative years. In effect we have children who already have fundamental biochemical and neurological issues to begin with, and now we are faced with the added difficulty of correcting the possible issues *while* these same issues make it more difficult to do so.

Perhaps the most important thing the current generation can do right now is to become more aware of the importance of the vagus nerve, and how it relates to one's growth and progress. If that can be done, then the future generations would be less exposed to the vagus-busting trends that so dominate the world today. We all want to raise a generation that is better-equipped to handle the world's evolving problems, and we could greatly increase our chances if we could raise a vagus-friendly environment for our children.

TAKEAWAYS:

- The vagus nerve plays a critical role in the physical and emotional growth of infants, along with how successful they will be in social situations as they grow up. The higher the vagal tone, the better one's chances of growing up without deep-seated socio-emotional troubles.

- Given this fact, vagus nerve stimulation should start at infancy, and vagus nerve assessment should be a part of every infant assessment.

CONCLUSION

If I had told you at the start that there is one nerve in the body whose activity effectively controls our destinies, perhaps you wouldn't have believed me. In fact, it would still be hard to believe up until now, if not for the wealth of scientific resources one can find about this topic. There is a huge body of research on disparate topics, all joined together only by the fact that the vagus nerve has something to do with them.

Perhaps it's a good time to really appreciate the wonder and complexity of the human body. Many of us had been taught of the body as a sort of computer where the brain is the central processing unit, the heart is the battery, and the lungs and gut the power cords connecting us to the power supply that is food, water, and air. But the human body is instead an intricate and highly organic system, where even the mighty brain takes cues from the rest of the body. Every organ system has a hand in determining the next steps for the body, and somewhere in that great switchboard of information, the vagus nerve sits trying to sort everything out.

This book has taken you through the whole gamut of research and details on the vagus nerve. By now, you should know pretty much everything there is to know about it, from its anatomy to its myriad of functions, from harnessing it for overall health to the issues that it can address in the near future.

But if there is one piece of info that you should never forget out of all that you have read, it is this: the vagus nerve is just a part of a network, a vast network of feedback and control, of input and assessment that we have not yet completely explored and mapped. With all these information on the vagus nerve, it would be so easy to spend all your time trying to stimulate your vagus nerve to its optimal tone. Now, all that's good, but it's still just a part of the overall equation of health.

Remember that the vagus nerve does not just relay information from the brain to the rest of the body. It also actively picks up information from the rest of the body, sending it up to the brain. While one can (in the light of all the research we covered) make the assertion that a person can only be as healthy as his vagus nerve, it would be more accurate to say that the vagus nerve could only be as healthy as the organ surrounding it.

You could have a perfectly functioning active vagus nerve... but you may still develop various illnesses thanks to your lifestyle choices. You may still be a victim of one of the GBDs. Note that while vagus stimulation can ward off certain issues, the vagus nerve is more or less just a mirror reflecting your state of overall health when it comes to other illnesses. It's so easy to confuse these two concepts. Stimulating your vagus nerve can't (at least not yet) cure cancer, but this cancer can show important signs when viewed through the vagus nerve.

In short, take care of the vagus nerve as much as you need — do the "bullet time" breathing exercises (or take a deep look at the contemplative traditions if you have time), fix your diet, do a routine vagal massage, and perk up your posture. But don't neglect the rest of the body, too. When you feel that something is wrong with a different part of the body, seek ways to cure it independently of vagus stimulation — but let the stimulation continue as a means of augmenting whatever other remedy you may use.

Observing the vagus nerve up close shows us a very important lesson, too. We are exposed to the idea that what we know about the slew of diseases affecting the world might just be the tip of the iceberg. With all the in-depth research we have, we are just gradually becoming more and more aware of just how interconnected things are, and how seemingly disparate things can actually be deeply related because of an overarching factor. Who knew that a reading in the EEG could predict whether or not you are likely to suffer from depression? Who knew that stimulating something other than the brain could help the brain repair itself from stroke? Who knew that the word "gut feel" actually has scientific backing, since the gut indeed talks to the brain? Who knew that the microbial flora in one's gut could even affect how moody a person can be?

One can only imagine the surprise of the first people who discovered the wonders of the vagus nerve. Today, that wonder lives on in the people who have had the opportunity to explore the powers of this twin bundle of nerve fibers winding its way through the human body. Just do a cursory search online and you will be seeing a lot of articles hailing the vagus nerve as the body's best kept secret to health, a holy grail of cures.

But again, be careful of such labeling. The vagus nerve isn't the holy grail — the human body, as a whole, is. We haven't even mapped the entirety of the vagus nerve yet, and science is still busy trying to find the best way to tame and stimulate it. But who knows if, in the future, we find some specific part of the vagus nerve — or a different part of the body, for that matter — that will concentrate all the nerve's powers into a smaller area? And then another one before that? The search for "the secret" will always continue, but never take your eyes off the fact that the body is a holistic system, meant to function as a whole.

Just like the meditative masters of old, may the knowledge you gained about the vagus nerve serve as building blocks on which you can build something synergistic — something that really is at one with the body and everything that is around it.

Thank you

Before you go, I just wanted to say thank you for purchasing my book.

You could have picked from dozens of other books on the same topic but you took a chance and chose this one.

So, a HUGE thanks to you for getting this book and for reading all the way to the end.

Now I wanted to ask you for a small favor. **Could you please consider posting a review on the platform? Reviews are one of the easiest ways to support the work of authors.**

This feedback will help me continue to write the type of books that will help you get the results you want. So if you enjoyed it, please let me know.

REFERENCES

Breit, Sigrid, Kupferberg, Aleksandra, Rogler, Gerhard, ... Gregor. (2018, February 1). Vagus Nerve as Modulator of the Brain–Gut Axis in Psychiatric and Inflammatory Disorders. Retrieved from https://www.frontiersin.org/articles/10.3389/fpsyt.2 018.00044/full.

Field, T., & Diego, M. (2008, September). Vagal activity, early growth and emotional development. Retrieved from https://www.ncbi.nlm.nih.gov/pmc/articles/PMC255 6849/.

Gidron, Yori, Deschepper, Reginald, Couck, D., Marijke, ... Brigitte. (2018, October 19). The Vagus Nerve Can Predict and Possibly Modulate Non-Communicable Chronic Diseases: Introducing a Neuroimmunological Paradigm to Public Health. Retrieved from https://doi.org/10.3390/jcm7100371.

Irena, Eva, Chládek, Robert, Martin, Jurák, ... Shaw. (2019, April 1). EEG Reactivity Predicts Individual

Efficacy of Vagal Nerve Stimulation in Intractable Epileptics. Retrieved from https://www.frontiersin.org/articles/10.3389/fneur.2019.00392/full.

Johnson, R. L., & Wilson, C. G. (2018, May 16). A review of vagus nerve stimulation as a therapeutic intervention. Retrieved from https://www.ncbi.nlm.nih.gov/pmc/articles/PMC5961632/.

Kitamura, K., Takata, S., Futamata, H., Teragami, T., & Hashimoto, T. (1997, August). Effects of head-up tilting on vagal nerve activity in man. Retrieved from https://www.ncbi.nlm.nih.gov/pubmed/9283229.

Lerman, I., Davis, B., Huang, M., Huang, C., Sorkin, L., Proudfoot, J., ... Simmons, A. N. (n.d.). Noninvasive vagus nerve stimulation alters neural response and physiological autonomic tone to noxious thermal challenge. Retrieved from https://journals.plos.org/plosone/article?id=10.1371/journal.pone.0201212.

Pereyra, P. M., Zhang, W., Schmidt, M., & Becker, L. E. (2003, March 14). Development of myelinated and unmyelinated fibers of human vagus nerve during the first year of life. Retrieved from https://www.sciencedirect.com/science/article/abs/pii/0022510X9290016E.

Yang, J., & Phi, J. H. (2019, May). The Present and Future of Vagus Nerve Stimulation. Retrieved from https://www.ncbi.nlm.nih.gov/pmc/articles/PMC6514309/.

Zhang, Y., Zheng, N., Cao, Y., Wang, F., Wang, P., Ma, Y., ... Feng, X. (2019, April 1). Climbing-inspired twining electrodes using shape memory for peripheral nerve stimulation and recording. Retrieved from https://advances.sciencemag.org/content/5/4/eaaw1066.

Manufactured by Amazon.ca
Acheson, AB